WELLNESS:
Small Changes You Can Use
to Make a Big Difference

WELLNESS:
Small Changes You Can Use to Make a Big Difference

Regina Sara Ryan and John W. Travis, M.D.

TEN SPEED PRESS
Berkeley, California

TEN SPEED PRESS
P.O. Box 7123
Berkeley, California 94707

Cover and text design by Nancy Austin
Typesetting by Recorder Typesetting Network
Illustrations on pages 5 and 139 by Ellen Sasaki

Library of Congress Cataloging-in-Publication Data

Ryan, Regina Sara.
    Wellness : small changes you can use to make a big difference /
  Regina Sara Ryan, John W. Travis.
       p.   cm.
    Includes bibliographical references.
    ISBN 0-89815-402-2
    1. Health.   I. Travis, John W., 1943–   .   II. Title.
RA776.R93   1991
613—dc20   90-19587
                                                                   CIP

Printed in the United States of America
     3   4   5   —   95   94

Printed on recycled paper

· · · · · · · · · · · · · · · · · · *Acknowledgements* · · ·

With deepest appreciation to Jere Pramuk who supports and celebrates my life. To Sue and Greg Bowser, Jackie Greenberg, and Meryn Callander for their gracious hospitality. To John Travis for sharing the labor and keeping the vision. Thanks to George Young, our publisher, and Jackie Wan, editor extraordinaire, for help and encouragement.

—RSR

Thanks to the thousands of people committed to wellness that I have met in the past 20 years, I can now say I know something about this broad field called wellness. To Regina for her diligence in crafting the words and to my "sisters" Joy Holloway and Bobbie Salzer-Rae for helping me keep perspective.

—JWT

For Mr. Lee Khēpā Baul (RSR)
For Meryn (JWT)

Contents

WELLNESS:
Small Changes You Can Use
to Make a Big Difference

Are you running more now, but enjoying it less?
Are you eating more fiber, but feeling more stress?
Are your thighs looking lean and your lungs feeling clean
But your kids seem more crazy than they've ever been?

And your spouse or your friends, are they sorely depressed?
Do they wonder why you are so madly obsessed?
Are your dreams filled with monsters of sugar and fat
While your fantasies plague you with nothing but that?

Are you tearing out hair in your frantic despair
As you worry what beverage to have with your fare?
Since coffee will leave you a jangling mess,
And cola will give your poor heart such distress,
And milk has been shown to contain D-E-S
Or whatever that stuff is that makes men grow breasts.

All the diets, the books about low-fat desserts,
All the threats of the cancer from non-cotton shirts
And the fears and the tears and the jogger's brassieres—
If you're not happy now, wait around a few years.
There'll be more things to worry about every day
And worse fumes to breathe in, and no time to play.
And I've heard even God's feeling not quite OK.

—R.S.R.

. . . . .

You are not alone if you are confused by the flood of data about health and fitness that fills the newspapers and magazines. Nor are you the only one who feels frustrated and unfulfilled even though you've been exercising vigorously, or eating "right" for years.

1

This book was written to encourage you to appreciate that, despite whatever confusion and frustrations beset you, you are not a helpless victim struggling in life's ocean, tossed by every wave. Quite the contrary. You are essentially in charge of your own life, if you choose to be, and possess resources of mind and body that are more powerful than you probably imagine. This book can help you to take charge of your life and health and to tap your inner resources in a practical and effective way.

In the forty-some years of our combined experience in the field of wellness, we have witnessed some remarkable improvements in health and the overall quality of life, both in our own lives and in the lives of people with whom we have worked. These improvements, built on a foundation of self-responsibility and greater self-appreciation, were accomplished with small changes—step by step. Unlike the more aggressive approaches advocated by many fitness programs or diet regimens, the kinds of small changes we support are usually quite gentle and simple. They are designed to increase self-awareness and presented in a way that will encourage compassionate acceptance of mistakes.

Small changes have a ripple effect because of the interdependence of all aspects of life. You can't wear tight shoes for very long before you start to notice that everything about your world feels cramped in one way or another. When you're worried about something, you're likely to have an upset stomach, too. What may appear to be separate events or individual symptoms are really interconnected aspects of a much larger and more complex system. So it is that small changes can have big results.

This book contains 32 simple "processes"—each one an entry point into the larger process of living healthier and growing in appreciation for yourself, others, and your environment. We call this whole process "wellness" and know that, once engaged, it tends to be self-reinforcing. For instance, learning to use a simple breathing technique to handle stressful events on the job may naturally draw attention to what is

---

A note about our pronoun usage: Throughout the book, we use the pronoun "you" to address you, our reader, both in a specific and in a general sense. We chose this word over the stilted "one," or the overly inclusive "we," recognizing that it may make assumptions that aren't necessarily true for you and that it may occasionally seem patronizing or condescending.

causing or increasing the stress in the first place. Before long, you may find yourself replacing your old desk chair with one that promotes better posture, and eventually replacing some tired old ways of working with some fresh and vital ones.

Every body is unique, and wellness prizes these differences. It is essential, therefore, that you learn to read and interpret the signals—both internal and external—that your body is giving you all of the time about what you need and want for balance, for healing, for greater vitality. Developing this self-awareness, in our view, may be the most important small change anyone can make. Self-awareness is the compass that will direct your path through the maze of health data.

There are no free rides or instant cures. Small changes, to be effective, must be practiced consistently over time. If you put your pocket change into your piggy bank every day, you will start to build a savings account for yourself. With that savings you establish some security. The analogy applies as well to your health concerns. When you master small changes, you build a fortified base from which to take further steps on your healing journey.

Wellness is not a state you achieve once and for all. There is no end point in this wellness process. And much as with every other process in life, it will have its highs and lows. You will make strides and live the positive results of those advances—in energy, strength, and vitality in general. You will also have periods in which you need to rest, to recuperate. What you are starting, or continuing, here is a way of life, not a series of prescriptions.

Wellness is not a limited or exclusive concept. Although many people associate it only with fitness, nutrition, or stress reduction, it is much, much more. Wellness is a bridge that takes people into realms far beyond treatment or therapy—into a domain of self-responsibility and self-empowerment. If you are ill, the wellness approach works alongside any forms of treatment you may be undertaking with your doctor or health professional, encouraging you to become an active participant in the healing process instead of a passive recipient.

We have divided the book into four main sections, loosely structured to take you quickly from basics to more advanced considerations within the field of wellness.

Part I, **Getting a Grip**, will orient you for the trip by helping you to remember what you already know and to set your goals for the results you want to have. It will supply you with a handful of essential tools you can use as you make this journey—like ways to handle stress and strong emotions. You will learn the art of "inhabiting your body,"

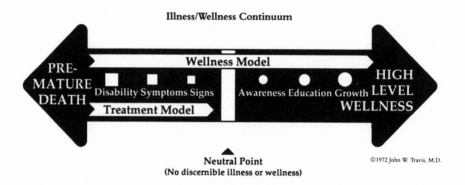

Illness/Wellness Continuum

Wellness Model

PRE-
MATURE
DEATH

Disability Symptoms Signs

Treatment Model

Awareness Education Growth

HIGH
LEVEL
WELLNESS

Neutral Point
(No discernible illness or wellness)

©1972 John W. Travis, M.D.

The Illness/Wellness Continuum. Moving from the center to the left shows a progressively worsening state of health. Moving to the right of center indicates increasing levels of health and well-being. The treatment model (drugs, herbs, surgery, psychotherapy, acupuncture, etc.) can bring you up to the neutral point where the symptoms of disease have been alleviated. The wellness model, which can be used at any point on the continuum, helps you move toward higher levels of wellness. The wellness model is not intended to replace the treatment model, but to work in harmony with it. If you are ill, treatment is important, but don't stop at the neutral point. Use the wellness model to move towards high-level wellness.

our phrase for how to develop self-awareness and self-appreciation so that you can become your own best friend, teacher, and healer.

Part II is called **Loosening Up** and it is designed to help you to gently and gradually stretch into your new choice for a wellness lifestyle. Here you will be invited and encouraged to lighten up through laughter, therapeutic touch, meditation, and other soft exercises, and you will be given simple instructions to get you started in the processes.

In Part III, we get down to the business of **Taking Action**. By now you should be limbered up and ready to initiate some of the processes that require a bit more energy or a stronger commitment—like starting an exercise program, or restructuring your relationship to food,

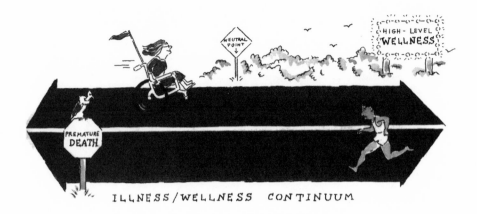

ILLNESS/WELLNESS CONTINUUM

Wellness is your right and privilege regardless of your current state of health or illness. There is no prerequisite other than your free choice. The "well" being is not necessarily the strong, the brave, the successful, the young, or even the illness-free person. You can be pursuing wellness and yet be physically disabled, aged, scared in the face of challenge, in pain, imperfect. Sound familiar? *What makes the difference is the direction in which you are headed.* Anyone can make some small change that orients them in that direction, and this book will show you how.

or building a support system, or changing your job. Not everything in this chapter will be useful to everyone, but there is surely something for everybody.

Part IV is called **One Step Beyond** because it moves you into areas that may be considered unconventional. Yet, in our experience, these areas are necessary for providing a more complete understanding of well-being. Perhaps you have never considered the powerful effects of music, sound, or silence in structuring a healthy environment. This section will inform you of the possibilities. You will learn how to create mental images that will relieve your stress and pain and even help you to heal faster.

Still want more? For those who wish to pursue this subject further, the appendices will introduce you to some of the more complex concepts that underlie our approach to wellness and will offer suggestions for how and where to make the next steps.

HOW BEST TO USE THIS BOOK

Remember, this book is a primer. It is a memory jogger, an inspiration generator, a referral guide. Use it as such and you will be using it to full advantage. Here are a few suggestions to keep in mind as you dive in:

1. **Begin at the beginning.** If wellness is new to you, we suggest that you work your way through the book to get the benefit of building more challenging processes on simpler and more basic ones. But since each of the small changes contained here is complete in itself, you can also jump in anywhere. Decide how you learn best and proceed that way. If you have a particular need or interest, check the Table of Contents to find the Processes that will address it.

2. **Be active.** This is a miniworkbook, not a novel to get lost in. Stay active by doing the exercises suggested. Engage us, the authors, by challenging and questioning whether our words are congruent with your own experience. Underline what you want to remember or want to study further.

3. **Ask for help.** Create a wellness partnership or a support system. Even if you are sure of yourself, or thoroughly trained in some health system, it helps to have someone else to share the healing journey with you—someone to talk to, someone to give you feedback or a reality check once in a while, someone to keep you encouraged, and above all, someone to care about you. So, whether it is a good friend or family member, a helping professional, or a support group, let yourself lean on someone else for a while.

   Think about who in your life currently supports you. Who can you rely on for comfort? For clarification or information? For confrontation when they observe you going off track? Who can you rely on for inspiration? Think about personal resources, like your friend down the block who can always be called in an emergency, or an acquaintance who works in a social service agency, for example. Many times people fail to ask for the help they need because they have forgotten how many resources they actually have. Make a list.

4. **Expect lots of questions.** This book is not about absolute prescriptions, specific diets, or regimented exercise programs, even though all of these things are considered. For us, wellness has much more to do with developing self-awareness—learning to trust your own internal guidance system through the information that your body is giving you. This is the key to creating your own vibrant life in your own way. That may take some serious question asking.

5. **Start a wellness journal or diary.** To write regularly about what you are learning by these small changes is a powerful tool for continued motivation. Our students and workshop participants are generally surprised with how much they know as soon as they start writing about thoughts and feelings. Writing helps to integrate separate aspects of wellness into a whole piece. As you put your practices and experiences into words, you are using another modality that will strengthen their impact on your life. Reading back over the history of your changing process will help you to chart your progress, and that will give you additional encouragement to keep it going.

   You don't need to limit your journal keeping to formal writing. Try using poetry, or drawing, or doodling to express what is happening for you. The books listed in the Resources below may be useful to you.

6. **Set short-term goals for yourself.** (See Processes 1 and 2 for help in this) Frequently evaluate your learning and reward yourself in healthy ways for your progress. Be open to modifying your goals as necessary. If you keep momentum in the direction of your original intention, something else might intervene and start you on another course that is even more desirable than your initial one.

7. **Take it easy on yourself.** Give yourself lots of slack (i.e., compassionate acceptance) as you encounter areas that need a lot of work and avoid compounding ill health or dis-ease by burdening yourself with guilt about what you are doing or not doing. Make mistakes and keep on going. It may be that you will start with a burst of energy but be unable to maintain that pace. Make each day a new beginning. Simply renew your intentions and practice forgiveness (see Process 28) for what you haven't done.

8. **Refer to the Resources** suggested at the end of each process to expand your understanding. We go into greater depth regarding most of the small changes covered in this book in our *Wellness Workbook*

(Ten Speed Press, 1981, 1988). The corresponding pages in that book are listed at the end of each process here. The *Wellness Workbook* is available at bookstores or by mail order (see the last page of the book).

Resources

Travis, J. and Ryan, R. *Wellness Workbook,* ix–xxxv. Berkeley, CA: Ten Speed Press, 1988.

Capacchione, L. *The Creative Journal: The Art of Finding Yourself.* North Hollywood, CA: Newcastle Publishing, 1989.

Rainer, T. *The New Diary: How to Use a Journal for Self-Guidance and Expanded Creativity.* Los Angeles, CA: J. P. Tarcher, 1978.

> IMPORTANT: If, as you are working with this book, you find that your problems continue to seem bigger than you are, it is *essential* that you get help. Don't wait. Seek out a helping professional or a support group that has experience with your particular problem—whether that is alcoholism, an eating disorder, depression, cancer, AIDS, or any other condition. Almost any hospital can refer you to professionals or groups that offer the type of help you may need.

Part I

Getting a Grip

If you were climbing a mountain you might need a trail map and a key to interpret the symbols used on that map. Here in Part I is the key to your trail map for the exploration of wellness. The processes contained here are designed to orient you in your initial steps towards wellness and will be your foundation skills, a collection of tools that you can carry in your knapsack and have available all the way. Welcome to the journey.

Use Part I to:

• remember what you already know about how to be well

• set goals for your wellness journey

• practice breathing for stress reduction

• appreciate the role of emotions in health

• simplify your life

• learn to honor the innate wisdom of your body

• reprogram yourself for health

• connect to the earth for healing and a healthier perspective

Start Here—
Remember What You
Already Know

· · · · ·

*W*ellness starts here, with the recognition that your body is wise, your mind is wise, and your soul is wise. You may not always honor that wisdom in yourself, but it is there nonetheless. You are at the leading edge of over five billion years of evolution. You are a being of amazing resources. It's time to remember that, again.

Humans have an insatiable hunger for answers and cures, and show great persistence in their searches, many of which have taken them around the world and back. Yet in looking "out there," they overlook, dismiss, and even demean the obvious—the knowledge that lies within.

Experts and guides are valuable in all aspects of life. But the trouble comes when all responsibility is shifted onto these experts, these doctors and teachers, and intuition and self-understanding are ignored. Giving away personal power to an ever-growing army of "professionals" puts one on the well-worn path to a power-robbed existence. Such reliance easily becomes a source of confusion when, as often happens, the advice of one specialist seems to contradict the recommendations of another.

· · · · · · ·

The next major advances in health of the American people will come from the assumption of individual responsibility for one's own health and a necessary change in lifestyle for the majority of Americans.

—JOHN H. KNOWLES, former president,
Rockefeller Foundation

· · · · · · ·

One simple way to practice self-responsibility is to acknowledge what you already know about your own life and health. You have a very basic sense of what's good for you and what isn't. By looking within and asking yourself some simple questions, you can access some of this information for your own well-being. If you are currently using a doctor or other helping professional, this additional information will be valuable to share with her/him. It will help to move you out of the role of passive patient and into a place of partnership on the healing team.

In a classic study conducted by psychologists Ellen Langer of Harvard and Judith Rodin of Yale, elderly residents in a nursing home were given plants to care for and were encouraged to do more for themselves instead of letting the staff take over all responsibilities. Another group of patients, of similar age and disability, received no such encouragement for self-responsibility. Within three weeks there was significant improvement in the health and vitality levels of the first group. Eighteen months later, even more dramatic improvement was observed. The death rate in the first group was half as high as that of the other.

This is only one example from a growing body of scientific research that supports the theory that individuals who maintain a sense of being in charge of their own lives stay healthier, live longer, and heal faster than those who do not.

An Experience in Remembering . . . .

1. Begin by letting yourself relax. Sit back and take a few slow breaths. Close your eyes, if you wish, to help achieve an inward focus, and just rest for a minute or so. Working quickly now, make a list of things that encourage your health and wellness. You can write out each response in a complete sentence, or simply use a word, phrase, or symbol. For instance:

   • **I know that more outdoor exercise helps me to work better.**

   • **I know . . .**

   • **I know . . .**

2. Next, make another list, this time focusing on things that discourage health and wellness for you. For instance:

   • **I know that eating in the car as I'm driving is not conducive to my digestion.**

   • **I know that . . .**

   • **I know that . . .**

3. Expand this self-remembering by writing yourself a letter about your current state of illness or health. Write as one best friend to another. Address any other issues that may be particularly troublesome for you at this time and don't hesitate to write about the changes you want to see and what you know will support you in making those changes. For example:

> **Dear Janet,**
>
> **I know you have been struggling for a long time with back pain, and I want to tell you I'm really proud of how you are handling the situation. There are some things that I can suggest that may be helpful for you, and . . .**

You will gain maximum benefit from the exercises suggested above by doing them periodically. For instance, try writing a letter to yourself every day for a week or more. Remember, as you write, that your health or illness is influenced by your state of mind, your emotions, your spirit. Consider these as you write your letters. You may find it helpful to write about your fears, your grief, your imagined weaknesses, and your negative opinions about yourself. Write also about your insights and intuitions, your dreams and plans, your day-to-day learning about questions of being and meaning.

Doing this kind of honest self-exploration will gradually reveal more of your own inner wisdom. This will give you confidence to trust yourself as the expert on your own healing. You can begin to shape your lifestyle in new ways that promote greater health and wellness. You can speak self-reliantly to your doctor, or other experts, about what you know about yourself.

Take that First Step Today . . . .

Now that you are off to a good start by remembering what you already know, it is time to act on that. Please don't discourage yourself by attempting an instant overhaul of all of your life patterns. Habits have built up over years and will take time to change. What is one step you can take today to encourage wellness? Whatever it is, write it down.

Do it. And give yourself a pat on the back for taking one small step towards health and well-being. For instance:

• **I will walk outdoors, vigorously, for ten minutes today.**

• **I will refrain from eating sugary snacks or desserts today and have fresh fruit or nuts and raisins instead.**

• **I will . . .**

Resources

Wellness Workbook, 1–21.

Capacchione, L. *The Creative Journal: The Art of Finding Yourself.* North Hollywood, CA: Newcastle Publishing Co. 1989.

Justice, B. *Who Gets Sick?* Los Angeles, CA: J. P. Tarcher, 1989.

Set Goals for the Changes You Want to Make

If your approach to life is mainly one of "going with the flow," you're liable to find yourself being washed down the stream, backwards.
—R.S.R.

· · · · ·

$\mathcal{T}$o have any real sense of getting somewhere, it's helpful to know where you're starting from and where you want to go. Goal setting is a dynamic tool for getting things done, and helps you clarify what is important in your life—i.e., what your priorities are. And, it aids self-esteem. By setting goals you are resisting resignation to the status-quo mentality that says you are a victim in life. Instead, you affirm: "I am responsible for my life and health" and "I am a worthwhile person."

Goals are like maps—they keep you on course. And more than that, goals are like magnets—they tend to attract things that help get them accomplished. It's almost magical at times, the way this works. When you put down in words what it is you want to achieve, you immediately start to see or remember the resources that are all around you.

Many people make lists of the things they have to do in a single day or week. When they cross some items off, they have a feeling of accomplishment. Even if they only get through half the list, they can still feel good knowing that they've moved forward.

There is power in setting goals, so tap into that power now.

Small Changes—An Exercise in Setting Goals · · · · · · · ·

Many times people overwhelm themselves by attempting to tackle a goal that they think they "should" have. They set their sights too high and then quit completely when they don't make the grade. It helps to make a distinction between the goals you *want* to have, and the goals to which you *will really commit*.

1. Read back over the letters and lists you generated in Process 1. Star any items that you really *want* to change or work on in some way.

2. Now look over that *want* list and put a double star next to any items that you *will* change or work on in some way at this particular time in your life. Write down those items in complete sentences that express your willingness to act. For example:

   I am ready and willing to commit to making a change in my habit of driving over the speed limit.
   I am ready and willing to . . .

3. Prioritize your *will change* list.

4. Starting with your top priority item, *brainstorm* for a moment or two about any preliminary steps you will need to take before you can start working directly on your goal. For example, will you need to purchase some special equipment? . . . shop at a different food store? . . . start reading a book on nutrition? . . . get some instruction in power-walking? . . . have a consultation with your doctor? Make yourself a plan and a deadline for accomplishing these preliminaries.

5. Next, go on to list the resources—people, places, things—that are available to help you in fulfilling your commitment. For example:

   My children—I can ask them to remind me of my commitment when they see I am breaking it.

6. Determine the length of time that you will work on this goal. An hour? A day? Two weeks? And decide how often you will check your progress and when you will reevaluate your goal. For example:

   For the next three days I will get up a half hour earlier each morning and take a vigorous 20-minute walk before having break-fast. I will evaluate my progress (how I felt during the walk; how that exercise affected my overall energy throughout the day) on the evening of the third day and decide then if I will continue the walks.

7. Keep encouraged by always congratulating yourself for any advances you've made, no matter how small. Remember, the bigger your

goals the bigger the challenge and the greater the likelihood that you will have setbacks. That's a normal part of growing and changing. Keep forgiving yourself for what you have not yet accomplished and honoring yourself for what you have.

8. Work on only one or, at most, two goals at a time. When you have established them as natural parts of your lifestyle, then move on to other goals.

Setting Goals for Life . . . .

At the same time that you are building your self-mastery by working on short-term goals, it is extremely helpful to map out a bigger picture for yourself—a plan for your life and health for years into the future. The exercise that follows will guide you in this process.

1. Take four blank sheets of paper. Head them as follows: 1) Where/ how I want my life and health to be five years from today; 2) Two years from today; 3) Six months from today; 4) How I would spend the next six months if I knew for sure they would be my last.

   As you work on these lists, be creative. Ask yourself: "What would I have/do/be if I had no limitation (like time, money, children, etc.)?" Work on each sheet as quickly as possible, taking no more than 15 minutes for each.

2. Read over all you have written and look for goals that are repeated or strongly expressed. These will be your priorities.

3. Put the exercise aside for a few days and then repeat step 1. Compare the results, looking for the goals that were clearly priorities in both writings. This exercise is designed to help you reveal your values and plan the next steps in your life journey.

4. Focus on one or more of your strongest goals and create a "road map"—a series of action steps that will bring your dream into form within the desired time. For example: If your goal is to be 35 pounds lighter and have a strong body in two years, begin by planning what type of exercise program you will use; when you will start it; when you will modify your diet; how much weight you intend to lose by the end of the first six months; and so on. Even the simple step of taking a trip to the library to get a book on nutrition or making a phone call to a local gym will be a good way to start.

5. Plan for frequent reviews and reevaluations as necessary to ensure that your steps are realistic and to keep yourself encouraged all along the way.

6. Share your goals with a friend and invite her/his support in helping you to stay on task, or join a support group that has similar goals. Creating a support network is invaluable to your journey. In fact, it may be essential.

. . . .

Approach those "impossible" goals by breaking
them down into possible increments. Or, to put it
another way: How do you move a mountain?
One rock at a time.

. . . .

TRAPS TO AVOID

Hundreds of different mental messages, doubts, and fears will arise to discourage you from designing goals in the first place and from sticking with them when you hit your first temporary setback. Some of these messages might include:

- "I already tried this once, and it didn't work."

- "People are always trying to get me to set goals. I'll show them who's boss!"

- "What if I set a goal and then don't make it? I'll feel worse."

- "What if I do make it? Will people expect me to do it all the time?"

- "It's a waste of time to make plans. Nobody can predict the future. Just take whatever comes."

These messages are dangerous because each of them is partially true. Of course you can't predict the future. And people probably will expect more of you if they see you are a person who can achieve a goal. But these messages can become self-defeating if you give them energy. Remember that they are only thought forms. Don't let them stop you. Keep moving ahead. The difference between a life of greatness and a life of mediocrity is that the great move ahead *with* their limitations, while the mediocre stay stuck in them.

Resources

Wellness Workbook, 198–200.

Covey, S. *The Seven Habits of Highly Effective People.* New York: Simon and Schuster, 1990.

Lakein, A. *How To Get Control of Your Time and Your Life.* New York: Peter A. Weyden, 1973.

Sher, B. *Wishcraft.* New York: Ballantine Books, 1983.

Handle Your Stress— with Breathing

· · · · ·

*U*se this process to start paying attention to your breathing as a form of relaxation, stress reduction, and healing. For additional help with stress reduction, see Processes 9, 11, 13, 14, 15, and 26.

Stress is inevitable—you need it to stand upright against the force of gravity. That's known as *eustress,* or positive stress, the kind that motivates you to get a job done on time or to do something that you thought was impossible. Endangered from without, or by disturbing thoughts from within, the body reacts to protect itself. It triggers off a set of automatic responses, including increases in the heart rate, in blood flow to the muscles, and in rate of breathing. These responses are designed to energize the body to do battle or to run away. When the danger is real, the alarm state is necessary and important.

But there are many other forms of stress in your life that have the potential of wearing you down and causing a variety of health problems. Many people live in a constant state of alarm. "Stress plays some role in the development of every disease," writes Hans Selye, MD, in his classic work, *Stress Without Distress.*

If stress is balanced by relaxation or attitude change methods, the continual surge of energy supplied by the stress-response can be modified or even channelled for creative purposes. If it is not, disease and breakdown will often result.

Take a moment to recall some of the stressful situations in your life. Difficult people—adults or children? Interruptions when you're trying to work or rest? Too much work, too little time? Driving in traffic? Smog and noise? Worries about your own health, or the health of someone in your family?

You may not be aware of it, but every tense situation, or even memories of tense situations, will cause a change in breathing. Generally, the more stressed you feel, the more shallow your breathing will become. People who are under the strain of a serious loss frequently report that the chest feels locked, like they can't take a full breath. That is why almost every approach to relaxation and stress management utilizes a focus on or attention to breathing.

Breathe to Relax . . . .

Here's an exercise that only takes a minute or so to complete, and you can do it imperceptibly almost anywhere, at any time.

1. If you can safely close your eyes, do that first. Otherwise, just stop talking and attend to your breathing for a moment or two.

2. Inhale, and as you inhale, say to yourself: *"I am . . ."* Exhale, and as you exhale, say to yourself: *". . . relaxed."*

3. Continue repeating, *"I am . . ."* with each inhalation; *". . . relaxed"* with each exhalation. Let the breathing gradually become a little deeper, a little slower, but don't force it in any way. Just watch it happening. As your mind begins to wander, gently bring it back to the awareness of breath and your statement, *"I am . . . relaxed."* Be easy on yourself. Continue doing this for a minute or two, longer if possible. Notice the overall effects of relaxation throughout your body.

MORE ABOUT BREATH

Adult humans normally breathe at the rate of one breath every six to eight seconds and inhale an average of 16,000 quarts of air each day. If nothing is done to restrict the breathing, it will happen naturally and fully. But people continually inhibit natural breathing in many ways—poor posture, tight or binding clothes, "speed-eating," exposure to noxious substances, smoking, and lack of exercise, plus habitual patterns of emotional stress all have a negative effect.

When breathing is obstructed or suppressed, the cells in the body do not receive the full amount of oxygen necessary to carry out their assigned functions. You may start to feel sleepy or irritable, or develop a headache. One of the reasons that exercise is so valuable is that it forces you to breathe more fully, literally replenishing your dwindling supply of oxygen.

Hindus call it *prana*—the life force carried in the breath. In many languages the word for breath and spirit, or life force, are the same. In

. . . . . .

The breath is life.
That is why the yogi says that you "half-live"
because you "half-breathe."

. . . . . .

Hebrew, the word for soul or spirit is *rauch*. In Greek, it is *pneuma*. In Latin, *spiritus*. Each of these words also means "breath." In English, to inhale is to "inspire"—to take in the spirit. To exhale, or expire, means to release the spirit. All of life can be observed as a taking in, and a giving out, of movement and rest, of controlling and letting go. The way you breathe is an excellent metaphor for the way in which you live your life.

Experience a Full Breath . . . .

While it is not possible or necessary to fully expand the lungs with every breath, to heighten awareness, it is vital to experience what a complete breath feels like. Taking a full breath periodically utilizes the lungs to capacity and extracts great amounts of "life force" from the air.

Try this exercise sitting, standing, and lying down. With gentle practice you will achieve a smooth and balanced inhalation and exhalation. Beginners should do it two or three times continuously.

1. Exhale deeply, contracting the belly.

2. Inhale slowly, expanding the belly first, then the chest, and finally raising the shoulders up toward your ears. Hold for a few comfortable seconds.

3. Exhale in reverse pattern, slowly. Release shoulders, relax chest, contract the belly.

Breathing for Healing . . . .

Conscious breathing practices are now routinely taught in childbirth preparation classes. Pain is intensified by anxiety, and the normal reaction is to then tighten up the breathing. Breathing consciously will not only relieve tension and help quiet the fear, it will also often relieve the pain. More and more parents are teaching breathing methods to

21

their children and using them when the child is feeling sick or scared. So, before you reach for the aspirins, the antacid tablets, or the telephone to call your doctor, do some breathing.

1. Scan your body mentally, noticing how different parts of you are feeling.

2. As you inhale, imagine that you are breathing increased life into areas that feel tired, painful, tight, or "starved" in some way.

3. As you exhale, imagine that the tiredness, the pain, the tightness, etc., are leaving with the expelled air.

4. Repeat for two or three minutes. Enjoy.

Resources

Wellness Workbook, 25–40.

Benson, H. *Beyond the Relaxation Response.* New York: Times Books, 1984.

McKay, M., Davis, M., et al. *The Relaxation and Stress Reduction Workbook.* San Francisco, CA: New Harbinger Publishers, 1988.

Befriend Your Feelings

· · · · ·

$\mathcal{P}$ainful or confusing emotions are par for the course in any situation of change—even a positive, life-affirming change in the direction of overall health and well-being. If you are using this book to deal with a present illness or disease condition, you are even more likely to encounter strong or disturbing emotions. Anger, fear, unexpected tears, feelings of abandonment and insecurity—all of these are natural and normal and necessary in any period of questioning or transition. If you have had surgery or are taking medication, emotional fluctuations are even more common.

The wellness process is a feeling process, but it is not always easy to plot the link between actions and the emotions they trigger. There may seem to be no logical connection between practicing a new breathing exercise, for instance, and a feeling of sadness that washes over you like a wave. Since there is no way to separate body from mind from emotions, any small change has the potential of arousing feelings.

In order to move into something new, you must let go of something old. "Letting go" is one way to describe loss, and loss is always accompanied by grief, however slight. When you stop smoking, you may feel the loss of that special rendezvous you had every morning with your fellow smokers. If you change your diet, you may feel resentment at watching others indulge freely in foods that you now avoid. Confronted with a life-threatening illness or condition, many people suffer great remorse for not having taken better care of themselves. Feelings are part and parcel of a life undergoing change. Be assured. You are not going crazy. You are probably right on schedule.

WHAT'S THE PROBLEM WITH FEELINGS?

In many cultures there is a great deal of confusion about feelings—especially the strong or painful ones. TV and movies portray people expressing themselves passionately and violently, but in everyday life there isn't much permission to rock the emotional boat. It is often considered a sign of weakness to display fear or grief overtly. The desired countenance is one of strength and control, so children are taught, at least by example, to be brave, to act "cool." People are very uncomfortable when those around them "break down." Others think there is something wrong with them when they feel depressed.

The cultural norms about anger are really confusing. People have come to expect the exchange of angry words in public and even applaud it as a motivator to sports and competition and war. The same people then express horror when battering and other forms of abuse are discovered to be rampant in families. Anger has become like a garbage can, in that many people use it as the way to eliminate any emotional energy that they don't know what to do with.

Joy and exuberance are generally acceptable as long as they are "controlled." It's all right to sing in church or to dance at a party or nightclub. But you might be thought crazy if you burst into song in a department store or danced ecstatically in the town square. There are many unwritten rules about expressing feelings.

Stop for a moment and recall some of the messages you got about feelings when you were young. What was held up to you as model behavior? Do any of these statements sound familiar?: "Don't get too excited, or silly, somebody's bound to get hurt." "Don't cry. That's for babies." "Don't ever say you hate anyone." "Keep going, no matter how bad you feel." "Just think happy thoughts and everything will be fine." "Don't expect anything, and you won't be disappointed." It is little wonder that many people have grown up to be emotionally confused and wounded adults.

There is a heavy price to be paid when feelings are denied or repressed. Lethargy, boredom, and a sense of deadness towards life may be the sorry consequence. When this happens, bigger and stronger forms of stimulation are required. Some people drink, others drive recklessly. Paradoxically, some people get seriously ill as a way to get attention and still feel alive.

Those who are unaccustomed to dealing with feelings in healthy ways often seek out other means to cover them over, or to distract themselves. At the first inklings of pain, fear, or loneliness, they may turn to alcohol, food, drugs, TV, unhealthy relationships, or compulsive work. Thus, bigger problems, more pain, and more fear are created in the terrified attempt to avoid pain and fear.

Repressing emotions out of fear or pain may lead to a habit of trying to control and dominate others as well. This form of relating—the uptight teachers who won't tolerate the enthusiasm of children; the rigid bosses who only want things done in their way—has, in some domains, become the norm. These highly controlled individuals, however, are emotionally unwell. Inner strength and integrity come with the ability and willingness to express emotions freely, to use emotional energy constructively. What that looks like is partnership, rather than a dominant or submissive role in relationship to others.

In considering the connection between wellness and feelings, we have seen over many years of working with clients and students what happens when "feeling" energy—anger and sadness in particular—gets blocked. Depression is common with those who do not allow themselves to experience rage or grief. And depression will weaken the immune system, making the whole body more susceptible to disease. Other people literally create a body armor by severely tightening muscles in their attempt to defend against painful emotions. Such armored bodies are more apt to develop symptoms of chronic pain and crippling disease.

How to Deal with Feelings . . . .

- **Adopt the attitude that feelings are natural and normal,** even if you are uncomfortable with them. This is a primary healing attitude. Strong feelings are not indicators of something "bad." Feelings have no morality. They just are. Accept strong emotions as valuable feedback telling you that something is in need of attention. And the best attention is gentle acceptance. Befriend the emotional parts of yourself.

- **Write about your feelings.** Express and explore them on paper. Write an angry letter and then tear it up, or compose a poem about your grief. There are many books that suggest ways to use writing for self-help. See the resources listed below.

- **Draw or paint or dance your feelings.** This is a healthy way to defuse potentially explosive emotions and to soothe painful ones. When you've expressed yourself creatively you may have a whole new perspective on the situation and may be in a more balanced place from which to speak to others.

- **Exercise vigorously.** Exert yourself. Exercising, even brisk walking, will take the emphasis off the worrying mind and encourage fuller breathing, which is a powerful healer of emotional wounds. Try digging a hole and speaking your emotional pain into that hole. Then, when you are finished, fill the hole with soil again. Let the earth carry your pain.

- **Talk about your feelings.** If you are confused, you can always start a conversation with a friend by saying: "I am not sure what I'm feeling," and proceed from there. Your listeners may not have answers for you, but the process of speaking opens the door for both clarification and support.

- **Change your mind.** Because thoughts arouse feelings, if you change what you are focusing on or thinking about, your feelings will change accordingly. When you are feeling frightened or inadequate, you can remember a time when you were strong and competent and create a mental image to support that. This type of imagery is used in many healing disciplines. (See Process 7 and Process 29 for practice in this.)

- **Surrender your feelings.** Give them over, along with the rest of your life, to a higher power.

Awareness and Acceptance of Emotions . . . .

Here is a simple exercise that will help you to sensitize yourself to how and where emotions affect your body, and encourage you to accept emotions as natural expressions of your being. You can do this exercise alone or invite a friend to help you.

1. Sit or lie down in a comfortable place. Close your eyes and breathe slowly and deeply to help yourself relax.

2. Repeat the following phrases five times each, very slowly but energetically, so that you can really generate the mood of the phrase. (Or ask your friend to say them for you.) As you speak, focus all of your attention on the physical sensations that these words evoke.
   - I am scared.
   - I give up.
   - I hate you.
   - I love you.
   - Please don't leave me.
   - No/no/no.
   - Yes/yes/yes.
     Add an emotionally charged phrase of your own.
     Try to sense where these various emotions "live" in your body and how they affect you physically.

26

3. Repeat the exercise, but this time let the feelings come and go as if they were currents of air that are just blowing through you. You can learn to feel your feelings without identifying with them so closely that they overpower you. Let fear *be there*. Let discouragement *be there*. Don't try to chase them away. Look at them. Then move on to the next emotional statement.

4. Share with your friend, or write about, what you have learned as a result of doing this. The more you "talk" about feelings, the more natural it becomes to accept them.

Resources

Wellness Workbook, 109–27.

Powell, J. *Why Am I Afraid to Tell You Who I Am?* Chicago, IL: Peacock Books, 1969.

Rainer, T. *The New Diary: How to Use a Journal for Self-Guidance and Expanded Creativity.* Los Angeles, CA: J. P. Tarcher, 1978.

Viscott, D. *The Language of Feelings.* New York: Pocket Books, 1976.

· · ·PROCESS 5 · · · · · · · · · · · · · · · · · ·

Becoming a Beginner—
Simplify

I like to live always at the beginnings of life . . .
I am by nature always beginning . . .
—ANAIS NIN

· · · · ·

*B*ecoming well in body and mind and spirit is not nearly as difficult as it may seem. Ageless wisdom teaches that only when one is experiencing life simply, and celebrating its ordinariness, is one living in harmony. In contemporary times, the Zen master and scholar, Suzuki Roshi has termed this approach to life the "beginner's mind."

Wellness is not a matter of accumulating something—like more data, or more special programs. Rather, wellness is realized by unburdening yourself of all that prevents the natural state of basic healthiness from being present. To be well is to become more simple.

How to Begin to Be a Beginner · · · · · · · · · · · · · · ·

- **Simplify your stuff.** How can you expect newness, freshness, surprises when every square inch of space in your home, and every corner of your mind is filled with "stuff" ? Give it away, sell it, or forget it. Leave room for something mysterious to take its place.

- **Simplify your diet.** Develop your taste for natural, whole foods that are cooked simply or eaten raw. Refining your diet in this way will have profound effects on the quality of your entire life.

- **Simplify your life.** Look carefully at all the ways in which your energy is being used, and note especially where and how it is being drained away. Say yes when you mean yes and no when you mean no. (See Process 21.) And remember that if you always speak as truth-

28

fully as you are able to, you will not have to worry about what you said.

- **Take time to rest your mind.** Use nature as a source of healing, and meditation or prayer as a daily practice for keeping attuned to what is most important. When the big picture is kept in the forefront, the little things just fall into line.

- **See your loved ones as brand-new everyday.** After living with people for years, adults or children, it is easy to develop the notion that you really know them. And in some ways you do. Yet it is a trap to always anticipate their reactions to certain things. Doing that almost assures that you will get just what you have expected. Acknowledge that human beings are much more complex and mysterious than that. There are always surprises to be uncovered, always new depths of appreciation that can be explored. Allowing someone else to be brand-new may start with pretending/imagining that you are meeting them, again, for the very first time. It works.

- **Watch your language, and your thoughts.** Expressions like: "I'm too old for that . . ." should be red flags, signalling you to become a beginner again.

- **Turn problems upside down,** especially health problems. Instead of assuming the attitude that problems are things to be fought against and conquered, try playing with the notion that an illness, or any other problem, may be a friend or a teacher at this particular time in your life. "Listen" to what it has to teach you, or what it forces you to practice—like patience, courage, creativity. A beginner won't consider problems as something "bad" or "good"—just "different" or "interesting." Admittedly this attitude isn't easy to hold when times are really difficult. It takes gentle persistence to turn problems upside down and to make this approach to handling upsets into a way of life. Why not begin?

An Exercise for Beginners . . . .

Look out the window, or step outside for a moment or two. Look at something, anything, in the natural environment—the sky, a cloud, a tree, a patch of earth. Soften your gaze, letting your eyes see each thing as if you have never seen it before. Be a beginner. Be an explorer. Let your curiosity about it grow. Now let gratitude rise. Imagine that this is the very first and the very last time you will ever experience this gift. Absorb the impressions as fully as possible with all your senses and let yourself feel gratitude.

The Hebrew word *dayenu,* meaning "it is enough," captures the essence of what it means to live in gratitude for life. To live *dayenu* as a way of life is to be ready to embrace the mystery of the moment, fully, and then to let it go. In this moment, all is like a gift given, undeserved. One breath is precious, one smile, one day of seeing the sun. If there is no next moment, this attitude allows one to die freely, happily, with deep appreciation for all that has been and is.

. . . .

The misery here is quite terrible; and yet, late at
night . . . I often walk with a spring in my step
along the barbed wire. And then time and again, it
soars straight from my heart—I can't help it, that's
just the way it is, like some elementary force—
the feeling that life is glorious and magnificent,
and that one day we shall be building
a whole new world.

—ETTY HILLESUM, 1942, Dutch Jew,
who died at Auschwitz.

. . . .

Resources

Wellness Workbook, 209–26.

Elgin, D. *Voluntary Simplicity.* New York: William Morrow, 1981.

Hillesum, E. *An Interrupted Life,* New York: Washington Square Press, 1985.

Steindl-Rast, D. *Gratefulness, The Heart of Prayer.* New York: Paulist Press, 1984.

Suzuki, S. *Zen Mind, Beginner's Mind.* New York: Weatherhill, 1970.

Inhabit Your Body and Love It

· · · · ·

*T*wenty-four hours a day your body-mind is talking to you—giving you feedback about what it needs for its survival, its pleasure, its growth, and its balance. Many of those messages go unnoticed or unheeded because of ignorance or lack of appreciation, or simply due to preoccupation with other matters. To inhabit the body means to start listening to what it is saying to you and learning to trust what you hear.

Few people escaped it as infants and toddlers—those wrinkled noses and the comments of parents about the "mess" as the diapers were changed. Perhaps you were admonished, "Don't touch yourself," and wondered at the concern this brought from your mom or dad. Undoubtedly it was drummed into you to keep yourself clean: "Scrub those hands; wash that hair; brush those teeth." Obviously the body was a pretty "dirty" thing! It wasn't to be trusted either. You were supposed to go to bed even when you didn't feel tired, to eat even when you weren't hungry, to wear a coat even when you weren't cold. If you weren't especially discouraged about your body's functions and the correctness of its feedback, you probably weren't exactly encouraged either.

It's not surprising that most people developed some dissociation from, and fear of, their own precious bodies and their natural processes. And, typically, that dissociation has endured throughout life. Even though the cultural norm encompasses an obsession with the appearance of the body, few people know much about the body's workings. When was the concept of innate bodily knowledge or wisdom ever spoken?

This shame and ignorance and dissociation, once learned, shows up as:

• overweight

• underweight

• obsession with the shape of the body

31

- seeming lack of concern with the shape of the body
- obsessions with cleanliness or tidiness
- fear of sexuality and intimacy
- physical symptoms like allergies, colds, headaches
- emotional deadness

To inhabit your body means to be aware of it, to listen to and learn from its constant feedback, to accept and feel all things—the pain and the pleasure, the happiness and the grief; and to speak about yourself as if you were a whole being, especially when some "part" is in pain. Disease is not the problem. More likely it is the body's attempt to solve the problem, a feedback of sorts that says something isn't working properly. And that "something" is probably lots more than a pain or an ache. These symptoms may point to the need for a change in life-style, for emotional expression, for spiritual guidance, etc. The only way to find out what your body needs is to inhabit it.

It is almost as if you live outside and a little to the left, or a little to the right, of yourself, but not squarely aligned. Rushing ahead, or lagging behind, or listening to others instead of yourself, or saying yes when you mean no—in these and thousands of other ways you check out on yourself. Wellness is about "coming home"—taking up residence inside your own body once again.

· · · · · · ·

If you want to know the secret of good health, set up home in your own body, and start loving yourself when there.

· · · · · · ·

WHAT INHABITING THE BODY DOES FOR YOU

- It tunes you in to the 24-hour-a-day feedback system through which your body offers valuable information on what it needs. You learn to "listen" to the body's reactions to different foods, different environments, different people. You learn where your weak and more vulnerable parts are. These are the places where disease first shows up. For some people that is in the throat. Others can literally feel the approach of a cold in the back and shoulders. Developing this kind of sensitivity to your built-in early warning system, you can often make interventions (like extra rest and liquids) that will prevent the disease from developing.

- When you inhabit your body you can't help but develop a greater sense of awe and gratitude about it. The abilities and adaptabilities of the human organism are incredible! Unfortunately most people don't learn appreciation for the body until something goes wrong with it. With heightened awareness, however, you may be inspired to start studying its processes more thoroughly in order to better interpret its signs. You just naturally want to take better care of yourself and to practice commonsense safety measures. You learn to accept yourself as you are—weak, in need, out-of-balance at times, a glorious series of contradictions. Honoring the body in this way builds self-esteem. This is your home. You are remarkable!

- Grace of movement is another advantage of inhabiting the body. You develop a more acute sense of where you begin, and where you end, and how far you stretch in any direction. You understand the relationships between head and feet and legs and arms as you walk and move around. You don't move unconsciously as much, or walk ahead of yourself, so to speak. Rather you move from the inside out, conscious of what you are doing.

- This sense of attunement to your own body encourages you to live in the present moment, to feel whatever is going on within you, both physically and emotionally, whether this is pleasant or painful. You taste your food and you experience your tears more fully. When you are so stimulated by your natural environment, you require less stimulation from unhealthy sources. You don't need drugs or alcohol to "turn you on" or excessive amounts of food to fill you up.

Meet Your Body . . . .

- Take a moment to remember, and look at, your feet. Realize that they have carried you, supported you, for how many years of your life? Bring your consciousness, and your feelings, into your feet. Touch them. Thank them.

- Put aside some time in which you practice increased awareness of your whole body. To start, take your hands and place them softly on one area of your body. Then bring your consciousness and your feelings there. Speak to this area. Thank it. Continue doing this for many areas—internal organs as well as external parts.

- After your bath or shower, let your routine of drying your body with a towel become a time to get reacquainted with yourself. For instance, be aware of your legs as you dry them. Slow down long enough to actually feel the texture of the towel against your skin. Imagine that you are waking up each area that you touch and experience the connections between all the "parts."

- Watch your language for ways in which you betray a sense of dissociation from, or hatred of, your body. Change your words from judgmental or condemnatory ones—"There goes that damn back, again . . ."—to simple statements of fact—"My back is painful." If these feelings of self-deprecation are consistent and strong, get help from a counselor or therapist.

Body awareness and appreciation is integral to the entire approach that this book takes. Refer back to this section as you continue working with the processes that follow.

Resources

Wellness Workbook, 15–16, 185–95.

Clarke, J. I. *Growing Up Again: Parenting Ourselves, Parenting Our Children.* San Francisco, CA: Harper and Row, 1989.

Houston, J. *The Possible Human.* Los Angeles, CA: J. P. Tarcher, 1982.

Trungpa, C. *Shambhala: The Sacred Path of the Warrior.* New York: Bantam Books, 1986.

Watch Your Words—
Avoid Illness Programming

The world is such-and-such or so-and-so
only because we tell ourselves that
that is the way it is.
—CARLOS CASTANEDA

· · · · ·

*T*he childhood rhyme that says "Sticks and stones may break my bones but words can never hurt me" is far from true. Words can literally kill. In the introduction to Norman Cousins's *The Healing Heart,* Dr. Bernard Lown, professor of cardiology at Harvard, tells a story that illustrates the power of words. A woman he was treating displayed severe panic-type reactions upon hearing the physician say that she had "TS" (tricuspid stenosis, a condition of obstructed blood flow in the heart). The woman interpreted this as "terminal situation" and reacted accordingly. She developed massive lung congestion and died from heart failure the same day.

Of course this is an extreme case. Nevertheless, it is true that your words create your world. As you look around the room now, you are talking to yourself about everything you see. Your language is structuring your reality. Furniture and pictures are not good or bad in and of themselves. They become beautiful or ugly, valuable or worthless, based upon your descriptions of them. The jeans you're wearing are fashionable or a mess, depending on your judgment of them. So too with your health. If you tell yourself that "starving a fever" will help relieve it, it probably will. If you say that arthritis and senility are inevitable, they probably will be. People tend to find what they have told themselves to expect.

Your brain operates like a highly sophisticated computer, storing each experience you have ever had. Brain probing reveals that subjects can describe minute details of events that happened to them as children;

clinical hypnosis allows people to remember things that the conscious mind may have filed away long ago. The body acts and reacts on the basis of its previous programming, even without the mind's acknowledgement. And so, many of your illness reactions and fears of today are the results of messages you received as a child. You keep these old programs in place by your unconscious self-talk and your mental pictures, and reinforce them with new input from contemporary sources.

WHERE OUR ILLNESS PROGRAMMING COMES FROM

- **Childhood role models.** You watched Mom or Dad start every day with a dose of aspirin for pain, or end every day with a few drinks to help handle stress. You wondered why certain topics—like sex and death—made adults very uncomfortable, and certain words—like cancer—were never used.

- **Direct commands from parents and others.** "You'll fall." "Oh, you'll get sick." "You'll cut yourself." And sure enough, you probably did!

- **Rewards for illness or for being in pain,** like special attention, touching, staying home from school, candy and ice cream, gifts.

- **TV, magazines and newspapers, advertising, billboards**—the media constantly supply direct illness messages such as: "The winter cold season is here!" "Don't worry about overeating, as long as you have those little white mints to fight indigestion." Even more insidious are the implied messages, like "Cancer is inevitable and will always mean death."

- **Daily conversations** with those who complain about their own symptoms and the ill-health of those around them.

- **Self-designed, self-destructive mental pictures of your pain or disease.** Humans are image-making creatures. Constantly and, for the most part, unconsciously, the imagination creates internal images of things that it cannot see (hear, feel, taste, etc.). Hearing the word "ulcer," you will form a mental picture (or some other internal sensory image—not everyone images *visually*) of one, even if you have never seen one. It may not be accurate, but the effect will be the same.

SELF-PROGRAMMING THAT HEALS

If negative messages and images can worsen a condition, doesn't it make sense that life-affirming messages will help to heal it? This is not just some fantasy. Current research in the growing field of psychoneuroimmunology is verifying what folk healers have known for centuries—that thinking and emotions have direct effects upon the strength of the immune system. It is the immune system that is the first line of defense against disease. If you can strengthen your immune system consciously, through the use of imagery and nurturing self-talk, you have a much better chance of maintaining the health of the whole body.

In the area of pain control, imagery and nurturing self-talk are used with great success. In a study conducted at the University of California, Irvine, many patients suffering from chronic back pain received long-term relief by using a variety of self-control techniques, including consciously slowing down breathing, mental imagery, and nurturing self-talk that reinforced pain-free feelings. Similar approaches are being used at many other pain centers in the US, and these techniques are being adapted for use in natural childbirth, surgical preparation, mental rehearsal for sports performance, and the treatment of burns.

Motivational programs and stress-management courses universally include some sort of training in the use of nurturing self-talk, or affirmations. These encouraging sentences should be repeated many times in the course of a day, and especially during times of discouragement or stress to counteract the effects of negative thinking and to inspire relaxation and build confidence.

You no longer have to be at the mercy of your own illness programming. By becoming aware of it, you will learn whether it is helping you or hindering you. You can then make some conscious choices. It is within your control to design new, healing images and practice choosing words that will support a healthier inner and outer environment.

Exercises in Reprogramming . . . .

• Start listening for your particular types of illness programming. Listen to how you talk to yourself about whatever you're doing or not doing. (For example, Regina noticed that after sitting at the computer for an hour or so, her lower back hurt. Usually she'd think/say something to herself like, "Oh no, I still have that bad back. What a pain. If it's this bad now, it will be a lot worse when I'm older." These negative

37

tape loops discourage, depress, and almost always disempower her by reinforcing the belief that the pain is inevitable.) Listen also for related voices of self-deprecation that tell you that what you are doing is not good enough, like: "You'll never win. You're all wrong. There you go again . . ." For a day or two, write down these messages whenever you notice them. Awareness is the first step towards change.

- Create a simple, nurturing affirmation that declares health and whole-ness, like: "I am growing in strength and self-mastery easily and peacefully." Repeat it morning, noon, and night, and whenever you notice the negative self-talk. Design your affirmation to address the particular issue that you most want to change by using this wellness program. For example, if you are working on eating more fresh fruits and vegetables, your affirmation might state: "I am enjoying the way my body feels when eating fresh foods. I appreciate myself for the care I show in eating more nutritious foods."

- Draw a picture of yourself being healthy and whole. Make several copies of this picture and put it around your house.

- Put cues in your environment, (like colored stickers or dots). Place them where you will see them often. Each time you spot a cue, re-mind yourself of your new programs and new pictures.

- Unplug your TV set and stop reading the news for at least a month. Notice any effect on your overall health.

- "Listen" between the lines to whatever you read, watch on TV, listen to, or talk about, to discover the hidden illness programs around you. Write them down.

Resources

Wellness Workbook, 128–47.

Achterberg, J. *Imagery in Healing.* Boston, MA: Shambhala, 1985.

Keyes, K. *The Handbook to Higher Conciousness.* Coos Bay, OR: Living Love Publications, 1975.

Miller, E. *Software for the Mind.* Berkeley, CA: Celestial Arts, 1987.

Rossman, M. *Healing Yourself.* New York: Walker, 1987.

Connect to the Earth

In wilderness is the preservation of the world.
—HENRY DAVID THOREAU

. . . . .

*T*he human body needs the touch of nature along with the touch of human skin. Yet too many people have dulled their senses and thus silenced that need. It's quite easy to go several months without ever touching the earth, walking on the pavement, moving from home to car to office to grocery store and back again. When was the last time you sat down on the ground or touched the earth in some way?

Physical contact with soil, natural waters, sunlight, and fresh air is healing. When stress has built to the danger point, a trip to the ocean or mountains, or even a walk around the block, is often all that is needed to restore perspective. Beyond that, contact with nature keeps you apprised of your place in the ecological system. In nature, you connect with forces stronger than the individual self, and this humbles you and puts the big picture in the foreground. Encountering other species that are more vulnerable than humankind similarly offers deep revelation.

Start Today . . . .

Here are some simple ways to connect with the earth again:

- Go barefoot, occasionally. Feel the grass under your feet; feel the sand; wade in the water.

- Grow plants or flowers to keep your fingers in touch with the earth.

- Keep living green plants and flowers around your house.

- Get outdoors, if only for a few moments a day. Let the sunlight touch you and warm you. (For longer periods in the sun, be sure to exercise appropriate care—wear protective clothing or use sunblock cream.) Even in the heart of a city it is possible to find green zones.

• Listen to the sounds of nature—the wind blowing, rain falling, birds chirping—even in the midst of an urban environment.

• Prepare your own meals using fresh and raw foods whenever possible, or bake your own bread. Carefully handling the fruits of the field keeps you aware of your connection to the earth.

• Practice the Navajo way of adapting yourself to nature, rather than trying to make nature adapt to you. As much as possible avoid dependency on air-conditioning in hot weather. In cold weather, keep the heat in your home at 68° F (20° C) or lower.

• When you are around young children, use language that communicates a healthy respect for the power of nature and a sense of awe at its beauty and mystery. Avoid teaching them that soil is dirty or that any creatures (even so-called vermin) are bad.

• Try to exercise outdoors as much as possible. Take a hike occasionally. Go for a bike ride instead of taking your car to the corner store. Roller skate in the park, or get a group of friends together for a ball game or kite-flying party.

• Plan your vacations for maximum enjoyment of the outdoors (with minimal environmental impact). Even a one-day family trip with a picnic can be a tremendously healthy break in your normal routine.

Resources

Wellness Workbook, 41–63.

Diamond, H., and Diamond, M. *Living Health.* New York: Warner Books, 1987.

Part II

Loosening Up

Too often you are challenged without being adequately prepared. It's like starting a run, or a climb up the mountain, without stretching your muscles first. Part II will help you with the
necessary loosening up. Here you will be guided in ways to
nurture yourself in preparation for the challenges of the path
ahead.

In Part II you will learn how to:

• make physical stretching a part of your everyday routine

• eliminate much of the unnecessary tension you carry around

• center yourself through meditation

• use water in many ways for healing and nourishment

• give yourself a healing massage

• take a break from seriousness and laugh more

Stretch Yourself

Stretching is the important link between the
sedentary life and the active life. It keeps the
muscles supple, prepares you for movement, and
helps you make the daily transition from inactivity
to vigorous activity without undue strain.
—BOB ANDERSON, *Stretching*

· · · · ·

One of the simplest and most effective ways to release tension and energize yourself is to take time out for a good stretch. You can stretch in almost any position, and, in fact, having a good stretch before you even get out of bed in the morning is a fine way to start the day. Developing the habit of stretching frequently throughout the day will make a big difference in how you feel.

Stretch yourself, right now.

Good.

Now take a deep, full breath, and stretch again in a different way than you did the first time.

Terrific.

Most people claim that stretching feels good. It helps release muscle tension almost immediately, and that results in an overall sense of relaxation. As it breaks up energy blockages in the body, stretching allows for better circulation. It improves range of motion, too. As you ease into a stretch, you literally reach farther. Stretching is an essential but often neglected part of a warm-up to any sport or exercise program because it helps in the prevention of injuries. It prepares the muscles for exercise, since a stretched muscle will resist stress better than an unstretched one.

Stretching is also a way to increase self-awareness. Focusing on how different body parts feel when they are being stretched increases your power of concentration and heightens your awareness of internal feedback. With growing self-awareness comes a greater sense of self-control. The more you honor the body, the more you "listen" to what it wants and needs, the more you will grow in awe of it. And this just naturally blossoms into self-esteem.

When you stretch, don't make jerky, quick, or bouncing movements. Instead, ease into stretches in a smooth, relaxed way and hold the stretched posture externally while you internally release the muscles. If you feel any pain, stop. Stretching that causes pain can lead to serious injury due to tearing of muscle tissues and loss of elasticity. "No pain, no gain" should be understood metaphorically, not literally, where stretching is concerned. Breathe consciously while stretching and imagine that you are actually breathing into the parts of the body being stretched. (Refer to Process 3 for instructions on fully breathing.)

A Morning Routine . . . .

Choose from among the movements suggested below or develop your own routine for starting your day with a stretch. Each of these stretches can be done in bed.

1. The rack stretch: lying on your back, with your legs flat on the bed and pointing your toes away from your head, stretch your legs as far as they will go towards the foot of the bed. Stretch your arms out to either side, extending and opening your fingers. Hold for a few seconds. Release. Repeat two or three times.

2. Lying on your back, reach for the ceiling. Extend and then contract your fingers. Tense, relax, shake your arms.

3. Still on your back, extend right leg over left leg at a 90-degree angle to your body. If this is not possible, go as far as is comfortable. Repeat several times. Then do the same with the left leg. Rest.

4. Bring your knees up toward your chest. Grasp them with your arms. In this position, roll to your left, then back to center, then roll to your right. Repeat as often as is fun. Release knees. Extend legs.

5. Still lying on your back, arch your lower back to a count of three. Hold. Repeat count and lower it to the bed again. Rotate pelvis clockwise three times. Rotate counterclockwise three times.

6. Bend your knees, placing your feet flat on the bed. Raise buttocks off the bed. Hold for a count of three. Lower buttocks back onto bed. Repeat three or four times.

7. Inhale as you turn your head to the right slowly, lowering your right ear to the bed. Exhale as you return head to center. Repeat, turning head to the left. Do this three or four times. Relax.

8. Roll over onto your stomach. Bend your knees and bring the heels of your feet back toward your buttocks. Hold. Lower feet to bed again. Repeat twice.

9. Bring your knees up under your chest, then reach back and hold your feet. Tuck head down toward chest. Feel your neck and back stretch with this one.

10. Let go of your feet. Raise head and straighten back, sitting back on your legs and feet. Look in the direction of the sunrise. Smile and greet the day. Get out of bed.

The All-Day Stretching Habit . . . .

Feeling uptight and depleted at the end of a day doesn't have to be the norm. You can use stretching exercises throughout the day, before and after every activity you perform, as a way of releasing stress, and as a way of getting back in touch with yourself.

• Driving your car today? Stretch before you get behind the wheel. Stretch as you drive. Take a deep breath and stretch your neck, your shoulder, your face. Adjust the position of your back frequently. On long-distance drives, stop every hour or so for a stretch breack.

• Office work? Try isometric stretches as you sit at your desk. Inhale, tighten the muscles in your arm, form a fist. Feel the tension mount from your fingers all the way up to your shoulders. Hold for a few seconds, then release completely. These exercises can be done with shoulders, back, legs, and the whole body. And they can be done so subtly that nobody around you will even know what you're doing (unless you want to invite them to feel better, too).

• Use everyday activities as a way of stretching out. Instead of mindlessly reaching for that box on the top shelf, imagine that you are doing a stretching exercise. Take a breath. Move smoothly. Hold the maximum stretch for a few moments. Try making your bed as a series of stretches. You can be creative and have fun, literally making a dance out of everything you do.

Hatha Yoga . . . .

The ancient discipline of hatha yoga combines slow movements and stretching postures with breathing exercises. Yoga is never supposed to be a huffing-puffing ordeal, and for that reason it is especially useful for the handicapped and the elderly, and for anyone who has not exercised in a long time, or who suffers from chronic pain. The postures not only stretch the body the way athletic stretching does, they also stimulate the nervous system and endocrine glands; activate circulation, digestion, and elimination; help to balance the energy flow in the right and left sides of the brain, and therefore in the rest of the body; align the vertebrae of the spine; and promote a deepened sense of inner peace together with grace of movement.

There are yoga exercises for every part of the body, from the eyes to the toes. Try this simple stretch called the Lion Pose, which is designed to relax tension you hold in your face. It feels great and looks silly, so it should make you smile!

1. Inhale.

2. While you forcefully exhale, open your mouth as wide as you can, stick out your tongue, and open your eyes as wide as they will go.

3. Hold this posture, without breathing, for a few seconds. Notice how your facial muscles feel.

4. Release the posture. Close your mouth and inhale deeply. The abdomen should expand as you do so.

5. Exhale slowly through the nose.

6. Repeat two more times.

Does your face feel warmer or more energized? Are you more aware of facial muscles that you never knew you had? Did you feel a stretch in other parts of the body as you did that pose with your face?

If you are interested in learning more about hatha yoga, refer to the books on yoga suggested here or contact your public library for videotapes or other books. Yoga classes are often taught at fitness centers.

Resources

Wellness Workbook, 96–100.

Anderson, B. *Stretching.* Bolinas, CA: Shelter Publications, 1980.

Bell, L., and E. Seyfer, *Gentle Yoga: A Guide to Gentle Exercise.* Berkeley, CA: Celestial Arts, 1987.

Hanna, T. *Somatics: Reawakening the Mind's Control of Movement, Flexibility, and Health.* Reading, MA: Addison Wesley, 1988.

Hittleman, R. *Yoga: 28-Day Exercise Plan.* New York: Workman Publishing, 1980.

Loosen Up Your Belt and Everything Else

. . . . .

*I*magine trying to blow up a balloon that is knotted in the middle and you'll have some idea of the stress created in the body when tight clothing restricts normal breathing. A tight and contracted abdomen, moreover, will adversely affect normal posture, digestion, and elimination.

Unfortunately, fashion trends generally are not motivated by the organic needs of human beings. "Figure-controlling" pantyhose, "all-day girdles," and tight belts and jeans are big business and not easily dismissed, yet they take their toll by fostering poor breathing habits. This, in turn, can result in a whole range of imbalanced conditions from hemorrhoids to circulation problems to headaches and more.

How can the diaphragm possibly do its job of expanding if the abdominal muscles refuse to move? The body will compensate by breathing from the upper chest, but the result is only a half breath. And tightness in the lower body will be exacerbated by the lack of oxygen flow to the area. No wonder you may feel sleepy or in pain after only a brief time of sitting at your desk.

Take a moment right now to mentally scan your whole body from head to toe. Be aware of your clothing. Feel tightness anywhere? Bra? Belt? Shirt collar? Necktie? Shoes? Now take a deep breath. Feel any areas of tightness or restriction caused by your clothing? How does your body feel, temperaturewise? Are you too hot? Too cool? Now, loosen your belt or any tight or binding clothing and take another deep breath. What are you aware of now?

Next consider your posture. Is it possible to breathe fully without strain in the position you are currently in? Where does the breath get "stuck," or, what parts of the body feel tight inside as you try to breathe deeply? Can you adjust your posture now to accommodate a full, relaxed breath? Do so if you wish.

BEYOND BREATHING

There is more to this issue than restrictive clothes and poor breathing habits. What about high heels, which are known to cause misalignment in the rest of the body? What about the position and design of office furniture, the height of typewriters or computer screens? These things can usually be adjusted to accommodate better posture or to give the body more room to move. Often people put up with unnecessary pain because they don't stop to think how easily they could change the situation.

Let's not overlook the issue of clothing fabrics and how these restrict the breathing of the skin. Many skin disorders and rashes are simply the results of irritation and improper ventilation caused by clothing. Popular synthetics, such as nylon, dacron, and polyester, are made of smooth fibers that can be very tightly woven. These fabrics are favored because they resist wrinkling. However, they are undesirable because they don't breathe. Since the body invisibly eliminates a substantial portion of waste products through the skin, open-weave fabrics like cotton and wool are preferable.

Many people need to wear a particular uniform or clothing style to conform to the dress codes of their jobs. But it is still possible to dress in healthier and looser clothing with careful shopping and a little creativity. Many shoe companies now carry styles that are sensibly designed yet suitable for business wear, and comfortable, neatly tailored clothing is available in natural fabrics.

Get in the regular habit of tuning in to your body, becoming aware of tightness or pain that builds up or surprises you as you go through your day. This tension can taken many forms. Some people walk around with their shoulders up around their ears; others keep the buttock muscles constantly contracted. You may wrinkle your forehead and give youself wrinkles and headaches; you may grit your teeth, and literally grind them down and create a chronic tension in the jaw; you may clench your fists, often to compensate for an unwillingness to express emotion in more direct ways.

And, besides trapping the tension in your body, all of these unconscious gestures expend energy. Start by becoming aware of how tightly you hold your toothbrush, or your pencil, or the steering wheel of your car. Over time, these unconscious habits can take their toll. They can hurt the body, as is the case with overvigorous toothbrushing, which can permanently damage gums. Sitting tensely behind the wheel of your car will increase contraction and pain in the muscles of your lower back, neck, and legs.

Loosen Up All Over . . . .

In order to appreciate wellness, your whole system needs to be relaxed and opened up and flexible. You need to be open enough to receive the energy that breathing and food and movement and light and human communication are offering you. It's hard to receive a gift in a closed fist. Once you have a better idea of your patterns of holding or contracting, you can consciously initiate the practice of letting go. In some cases you may need to visit a health professional who specializes in your particular condition. For instance, TMJ (temporal-mandibular joint) syndrome, a chronically tight condition of the jaw, can be helped with biofeedback training, among other approaches. But, for most patterns of tension, self-care is all that is needed.

- **Use your breath** to help in relaxing tense areas. When you notice that tension is present, consciously direct your breath into that part of the body. Imagine, as you inhale, that the oxygen is flowing freely, in and around the tense spots. Feel it loosening muscles and supplying renewed energy to the area. (See Process 3 for assistance in this.)

- **Use visual imagery** to release stored tension. When you find your shoulders (or any part of your body) tight, create an image that soothes. For example, imagine that you are standing under a warm shower that is softening the tough places or washing away the tension; or see yourself floating on a cloud. (See Process 29 for help in creating visualizations.)

- **Use self-massage.** You don't need to know any fancy techniques to release tension in your own body. If your face is contracted with worry or concentration, a few gentle strokes with your fingertips in the areas of tension can transform it. When you touch a part of your body consciously and tell it to let go, it often will, immediately. (See Process 13 for more suggestions about self-massage.)

- **Use self-talk.** It is possible to help alleviate the pain and tension caused by contracted muscles by simply repeating a soothing phrase. "My lower back is loosening and warming," for instance. The talk focuses your attention on the hurting place, and that attention catalyzes the relaxation of the muscles. (Refer back to Process 7 for suggestions about the use of healing words and phrases.)

- **Move the tension out.** Physical exercise is a great way to relieve overall bodily tension. Go for a swim or a brisk walk, or put on some music and dance. Pretend that you are shaking the tension off as you move. You will find that you actually are. (See Process 15.)

Resources

Wellness Workbook, 25–40.

Miller, E. *Software for the Mind.* Berkeley, CA: Celestial Arts, 1987.

Smith, P. *Total Breathing.* New York: McGraw-Hill, 1980.

Find Your Center— Learn to Meditate

The more faithfully you listen to
the voice within you, the better you will hear
what is sounding outside.
—DAG HAMMARSKJOLD

. . . . .

$\mathcal{L}$iving on planet Earth in the 20th century is stressful. You are bombarded by forces that push on you from all directions and leave you feeling unsettled and fragmented—making you more receptive to disease. It is easy to lose touch with what you really want, what you really believe, and ultimately who you really are.

In order to stay happy and healthy, you need a safety valve, a way to release excess pressure, a way to hold yourself together under stress. Many meditation forms are popular today because they are so effective in this. They aid in relaxation, concentration, and the attunement to deeper, more spiritual aspects of the self. Meditation is a process of locating your own center of being, your "temple" of inner wisdom, your truest self—and learning to live, consistently, from there. It is a form of recollection of your scattered parts. The word "meditation" itself comes from the Sanskrit word *medha* which literally means "doing the wisdom."

Begin to Meditate . . . .

1. Set aside at least ten minutes a day, and ideally longer, in a quiet and private place. (Most meditation forms range in length of practice time from 20 minutes to an hour.)

2. Be prepared to encounter thousands of mental distractions. Let them rise and fall or float away like leaves in a moving stream. Don't get washed away with them. Develop an attitude of passive acceptance.

3. Select a centering device. For some this will be a sound or word or phrase—a mantra—that is repeated. (For example: "One" or "Peace" or a phrase like "There is only love.") Others make use of a candle or devotional picture to keep the attention focused. Singing an in-spirational song, reciting a favorite poem, or using a repetitious bodi-ly movement like swaying or rocking can create the same centering focus. Concentrating on the breath as it rises and falls or simply counting breaths are other common forms of centering.

4. With many extraneous thoughts now removed from the mind, the body and mind are free to rest deeply. For some people this naturally evolves into a time of wordless gratitude. Others find that intuition or the inner voice is more clearly heard or perceived.

5. Keep bringing your attention back to the focus or center. As the mind wanders, and it always will, imagine that you are taking it gently by the hand and leading it back to the center—the way you might lead an exuberant child back to the sidewalk on the way to school. Let gentleness be the guiding principle.

6. Use resources as you need them. There are many books available that will teach you simple meditation practices. Use them to guide you. In many cities and on many college campuses there are groups devoted to teaching meditation techniques. Energy is greatly inten-sified when meditation is done with a group. You will be amazed at how many people secretly practice some form of personal spiritual practice like meditation. Start asking and listen to what they have to say.

Finding a center, a home, a place of balance within makes almost anything easier to face. The universe, from this perspective, is viewed as friendly, and your place in it is experienced as blessed. Since your life energy emanates from your center, being there regularly means being in harmony with yourself, your brothers and sisters, and with the cosmos.

. . . .

To love is to approach each other
center to center.

—PIERRE TEILHARD DE CHARDIN

Finding Center . . . .

People commonly speak about being "off center," meaning imbalanced in some way. This exercise is about finding an "on-center" place within your body, a place you can attend to when you are stressed or upset and need to draw your fragmented "parts" back together. This exercise is meant to help you find your built-in centering device that can be used throughout your day, no matter where you are, to help you feel at home again. Touch each place as suggested by the directions below:

1. If you imagine that your soul exists at some place in your body, where would it be? Touch that place now.

2. Imagine that your body is a building with a hidden chamber located somewhere within it. In that chamber you get to meet your inner wisdom or guide. This is a place in which no lies can exist. Where is that place?

3. Imagine that you want to balance your physical body. Where is the fulcrum, point of contact at which you will balance?

4. Take a few slow and very deep breaths. From what place does the breath originate? What place does the deepest breath reach?

5. Say "I am me" several times as you point to yourself. Where do you point? Which place feels truest?

You may have found several different places that felt like your "center," your "home." Decide which one is your favorite for now and experiment with it for at least a week or more before you try out another one. The idea is to use that place within as a point of focus that you can return to even in the midst of the most chaotic activity. Meditation then becomes a way of life, not just something you do for a set time each day. This form of self-remembering is a powerful means of heightening your awareness of your own life, reducing stress, altering the way in which you see the world, and consequently enhancing your overall health and wellness.

Resources

Wellness Workbook, 209–26.

Adair, M. *Working Inside Out—Tools for Change.* Berkeley, CA: Wingbow, 1984.

LeShan, L. *How to Meditate.* New York: Bantam Books, 1974.

Ram D. *Journey of Awakening: A Meditative Guidebook.* New York: Bantam, 1985.

Trungpa, C. *Shambhala: The Sacred Path of the Warrior.* New York: Bantam, 1986.

Drink More Water—
And Other Healthy Uses of H_2O

*If you could accurately assess your body's
need for water, you'd probably find that you
are at least two quarts low.*
—ANONYMOUS

. . . . .

$\mathcal{A}$ll humans come from the water: evolving from the creatures of the sea, bathing in the uterus of the mother. In reality, everyone is basically made of water, since water accounts for about 70 percent of overall body weight.

Water is essential to balanced health. The body relies upon it for digestion, for cooling, for elimination, and for the circulation of nutrients to every cell. Low-level dehydration is commonplace, and many people are unaware that this may be occurring for them, simply because they do not feel thirsty. So, drink up! Eight big glasses of clear water a day is a good recommendation to follow. Don't assume that you are getting enough water from the foods you eat and the beverages you consume. Many water-based drinks, like coffee and sodas, contain caffeine and sugar, which actually have a dehydrating effect. More water is required to aid in their digestion and metabolism.

Unless your system is flushed regularly from the inside out, toxins from food and air will accumulate in fat cells (everyone has them), muscles and joints, causing pain and stiffness and various health problems. Most kidney stones, for instance, consist of urates, phosphates, oxalates, and other wastes that have crystalized from urine that was too concentrated, rather than being excreted as dissolved solids. To protect against this kind of accretion, drink sufficient water. Constipation and headaches are often the result of insufficient water in the system. When feces are hard and small, and sink rather than float, this may also indicate that there is not enough water in the diet.

Drinking plenty of water is also an aid in maintaining your ideal weight, since water gives you oral gratification and a sense of fullness, no matter how temporary. It is possible that some types of overeating are merely the body's way of compensating for the lack of water it craves.

Because many urban water supplies contain traces of pollutants such as lead, asbestos, and mercury, which can accumulate in the body over time, consider using bottled spring water that has been tested by an independent laboratory (call or write the bottler), or attaching a high-quality filter to your spigot.

OTHER WAYS TO HEAL YOURSELF WITH WATER

Those with a history of heart disease or high blood pressure should check with a health professional before using the water treatments suggested below.

Now that you have considered water as a necessary part of your diet and a source of inner cleansing, look at some of the ways in which it can refresh and cleanse and heal you from without.

- **Showers.** Alternate hot and cold water as an aid to circulation. Showers are great for washing away the accumulated tension and worries of the day.

- **Baths.** Nothing beats a bath to help alleviate the soreness in muscles. If your bath is warm enough so that it causes you to sweat a bit, it provides the added benefit of helping to release toxins through the steam-opened pores of your skin. For relaxation, fill a tub with comfortably hot water and add a few drops of mild bath oil to moisturize the skin. Light a candle. Burn some incense. Take a glass of juice. Play some soft, slow music. Nurture yourself.

- **Swimming.** Regular swimming is a great form of aerobic exercise. Or you can exercise in the water to achieve similar benefits. Whether you know how to swim or not, it is therapeutic just to get in the shallow water and splash out your frustrations or problems. Be a child again—play!

- **Sweating** (in a sauna, steam bath, or sweat lodge) or **soaking** (in a spa, hot tub, or mineral springs). These ancient remedies for stress

56

and pain are as valuable today as they have been for centuries. If you can't get to a spa, soaking your feet in the bathtub or a basin at home is a simple way to enjoy and heal yourself.

- **Hot compresses.** Grate some fresh ginger root and wrap it in cheese-cloth. Place it in a large pot of water. Heat the water, but do not let it boil. Turn off the heat and soak a towel in the water. Carefully remove the towel; let it cool until it is comfortable enough to handle, then wring it out. Apply the towel to any ailing body part. Leave on until the heat is exhausted. Then do it again.

- **Rituals.** Compose a ceremony in which you use water to symboli-cally cleanse your body, mind, and soul from illness, darkness, "sin," and painful memories. This is a beautiful way to love yourself. Take a new or additional name to signify your forgiveness of yourself. Be at peace.

• •

Right now, go get yourself a big glass of water. Drink it slowly and experience it with all your senses.

Resources

Wellness Workbook, 47–49.

Watkins, R., et al. *The Water Workout Recovery Program.* New York: Contemporary Books, 1988.

Give Yourself a Massage, or Get One

· · · · ·

$\mathcal{T}$he skin is the largest organ of the body and accounts for almost one-fifth of total body weight. The skin is constantly growing and changing in sensitivity as it performs its many functions: protection, sensation, regulation of temperature, excretion, respiration, and the metabolism and storage of fat.

Touch is the first sense to develop in the newborn. As the infant takes its first breath, it reaches out to learn what its new world is all about. Sensory receptors located in the skin start picking up enormous quantities of information and sending them to the brain. Pressure, temperature, pleasure, pain—each stimulus carries a message about the environment. Each one adds another bit to the infant's store of experience.

For a baby to develop normally, it is essential that it be touched, physically handled. When touching is denied or severely restricted, an infant may actually die. Thousands of children in US foundling homes died until, in the late 1920s, this connection between touch and life was understood and remedied. Adults who were deprived of physical stroking in childhood often adopt compulsive, destructive habits such as nail-biting, overeating, or smoking. There is some speculation that violent behavior too may be a result of touch deprivation in early childhood.

Yet few adults appreciate how valuable touch can be. Many adults actually avoid bodily contact other than with a few intimates. If they weren't touched with care and nurturance as children, they may view touching with suspicion and fear. Many people even fear their own bodies and are reluctant to touch or massage themselves. They are not "at home" inside their own skin. Others were taught long ago that touching themselves was sinful, and those vestiges of fear still remain, especially in sexual expression. Because of the connection between touch and sex, they may be loath to touch others except in formal handshakes because they don't want their actions to be misjudged.

Those who are this afraid to touch or to be touched deprive themselves of a powerful source of nurturance and healing. In fact when they are depressed or anxious, there may be an even greater tendency to withdraw from the very things that would help to move them out of these states—the reassuring touch, the sympathetic hug, the healing massage.

While certain approaches to massage continue to remain suspect by the public-at-large, there is a growing acceptance of therapeutic massage even within the medical profession. In the 1970s, at the New York University Medical Center, Dolores Krieger, RN, PhD, conducted a study to determine the value of what she called "therapeutic touch." One group of patients received regular care, another group received a simple form of touch from their nurses, similar to the laying on of hands, twice a day. Within one day significant results were realized. The "touched" patients had increased blood hemoglobin levels (hemoglobin, which is found in the red blood cells, is what carries oxygen from the lungs to the other body tissues). The control group of patients showed no change in this aspect. In other test cases, Krieger has verified the value of therapeutic touch in accelerating the healing process. Patients experiencing this form of touch consistently report feeling profound relaxation and the alleviation of pain and other symptoms of stress-related diseases, such as nausea, poor circulation, and tachycardia (excessively rapid heartbeat).

As a form of nurturance and rebalancing, and as an aid to healing, massage is hard to beat. Besides, it's nonfattening, and if you do it yourself, *it's free*. Some of the positive results of massage include:

- relief of pain and tension

- improvement of muscle tone

- the maintenance of a healthy complexion

- release of emotional blocks caused by trauma and repression

- increase of blood flow and electrical energy to "wake up" tired body parts

- pleasure

- general balancing of right and left, and upper and lower parts of the body

Begin with Self-Massage . . . .

Self-massage is a type of self-care—a way to heal, to increase self-awareness, and to build self-appreciation (see Process 6). Besides, it feels so good and it's easy to do. You simply put your hands on your body and you start moving them. Lotions, special techniques, and formal training can certainly enhance the experience, but they can also lead you to believe that you need them to do it right. Not true. As you massage yourself, "listen" through your hands and let your hands accept feedback from your body and respond accordingly. The more you can quiet the chatter and judgement in your mind and allow your hands to move intuitively, the more creative, relaxed, and enjoyable the results will be.

Try a Head Massage . . . .

1. Remove glasses or contact lenses and turn down bright lights. Then rub your hands together to warm them. Slightly cup your palms, fingers together, and place them on your face. Hold them there for 30 seconds or so while you relax.

2. When ready, let your hands move over your face in a variety of slow or rhythmic movements, as you like: make circular moves with fingertips, follow contours of face with finger pressure, knead the skin, etc. Take your time.

3. Move your fingertips onto your skull and through your hair. Press all over. Try tapping or rubbing the scalp, or even grasping and firmly pulling your hair for additional stimulation. Explore other options for yourself. Be creative.

4. Stroke your head and face smoothly and gently all over, soothing your eyes, ears, lips, throat. Say nice things to yourself as you do this.

5. Using your fingertips, massage your gums by feeling them through your cheeks.

6. Gently and sensuously wash your face, or apply warm towels over it. Splash with cold water to conclude and apply some natural oil or lotion for a moisture treatment.

And a Foot Massage . . . .

The rubbing of tired feet is an age-old practice. In Oriental medicine, body energy, or "chi," is believed to flow lengthwise along energy meridians that end in the feet. Several contemporary therapeutic approaches, like zone therapy and foot reflexology, suggest that there are points on your feet that correspond to every part of your body such as the glands, or spinal column. The working of the feet is then comparable to massaging the entire body. The practitioners of foot reflexology believe that with pressure or massage energy blockages can be broken up in the feet, thus recharging the corresponding segment of the body. While many of these claims are not scientifically verified, the value of foot massage as a simple, loving, and therefore healing tool is undisputed by anyone who has ever received one.

1. Position yourself so that you can comfortably hold one of your feet in both hands.

2. Using massage oil or lotion, if you wish, start by rubbing your feet and ankles all over. Massage the heel, the areas between your toes, the top as well as the bottom of the foot, and your arch. Generally, wake your foot up.

3. With specific pressure from the thumb pad or the knuckle of your index finger, explore your toes and feet for areas of soreness and sensitivity. Gently massage those areas, using a smooth, circular motion for fifteen seconds or less. Then move on to another area.

4. When you are finished, rub your foot all over as if you were smoothing the skin. Stretch your toes and rotate your ankle. Then begin on your other foot.

Massage for Pain Relief . . . .

While acute or long-term pain should always be checked out by a health professional, you can help yourself with everyday pains and aches. If you can reach the part of the body that is in pain you may be able to relieve it. Using both hands if possible, cup them slightly and lay them over the painful area. Now begin to breathe slowly and deeply. Imagine that you are breathing warmth and energy through the hands and into your body at that point. Imagine that this warmth and energy flows into you through the top of your head and flows out through your hands. Sense that pain and tension are melting away under your hands.

Keep your hands in the same position until you feel a shift in your overall level of relaxation or a lessening in the degree of pain.

USE MASSAGE WITH OTHERS, TOO

All of the exercises suggested above can be done with a partner. Consider sharing the gift of touch with another person and allowing yourself to receive this gift in return. Again, it isn't necessary to have formal training. Your intention to offer comfort or relief is all you need to begin to make use of healing touch.

Resources

Wellness Workbook, 41–62.

Downing, G. *The Massage Book.* New York: Random House/Bookworks, 1972.

Kreiger, D. *Therapeutic Touch: How to Use Your Hands to Help or Heal.* New York: Prentice Hall Press, 1986.

Lighten Up with Humor, Play, and Pleasure

The weight of the burden is the seriousness with which we take our separate and individual selves.
—THOMAS MERTON

· · · · ·

$\mathcal{T}$he process of becoming healthier can be presented as such serious business that you can easily lose all the humor and joy in living that characterize well-being. So many of the books about health are filled with predictions of dire consequences for failure to follow a particular method, horror stories of what certain foods or lack of foods can do, warnings about the cancer-causing qualities of everything. It's enough to make you crazy!

Recent studies indicate that humor is an effective stress reducer and that it may actually increase antibody production, which means a stronger immune system. In 1964, Norman Cousins, then editor of *Saturday Review,* helped to heal himself from a life-threatening disease through a regimen of vitamin C, renewed self-responsibility, and humor. His reading of several classic books on the subject of stress convinced him that disease was fostered by the chemical changes in the body produced by emotions such as anger and fear. He wondered if an antidote of hope, love, laughter, and the will to live would have the opposite effect. Encouraged by watching Marx brothers movies and "Candid Camera" TV sequences, reading humorous books and stories, and hearing jokes, he found that short periods of hearty laughter were enough to induce several hours of painless sleep. Years later, Cousins recommended laughter to others, claiming that this "inner jogging" was beneficial in stimulating breathing, muscular activity, and heart rate.

The Laughter Project at the University of California, Santa Barbara has found that laughing is as beneficial as biofeedback training in reducing stress. Laughter, the researchers state, has its own unique advantages because it can be done anywhere. The only requirement is a funny bone.

Raymond Moody Jr., MD, the author of *Laugh after Laugh: The Healing Power of Humor,* has used this approach with his patients for many years. Humor works, he claims, because laughter helps take your mind off pain and problems, and catalyzes the basic will to live.

Take a Seriousness Break Right Now . . . .

- Look in the mirror and make the wildest, ugliest face you can make. Now make an uglier one.

- Throw away your troubles. Stand up right now. Form your hands into fists and bring them together at the center of your chest. Raise elbows on a line with your fists. Thrust elbows back, expanding your chest and drawing shoulder blades together. As you do this briskly for a minute or so, say out loud "Get off my back" and mean it! Release whatever is burdening you.

- Read the comics in today's paper. Forget the front page for a while.

- Put on a comedy video, if you have one. Cue it up to your favorite funny part and play it and replay it several times. Rent a few comedy tapes or go to a light, entertaining movie. Do this regularly. John's favorite laughter video is Michael Nesmith's *Elephant Parts;* Regina recommends *Harold and Maude.*

- Collect jokes. Ask anyone around you for a joke or two. Call a friend and have them tell you a joke, even if they know you've heard it before. Now you share one with them. Get silly!

- Watch young children or puppies at play. They're always good for a delightful laugh.

- Remember laughing so hard that your stomach hurt? Can you recall what provoked that? Let yourself feel it again.

. . . .

It takes a long time to become young.

—PICASSO

. . . .

REDEFINING PLAY

Play is an essential component of wellness. It is necessary to keep the fun-loving part of yourself alive, nurtured, and happy. The dictionary defines play as recreation. Re-creation! So, in the fullest sense of the term, it means to make new, to vitalize again, to inspire with life and energy. When you give yourself time to play you give yourself new life.

What words do you associate with play? Are they active words, like *silliness, craziness, sports, games, excitement?* Perhaps one of the reasons people don't play more is that they have accepted a very narrow definition of play. Maybe they've looked around at what society tells them is "fun" to do, and found that it wasn't.

Consider that play can also be described as absorbing, fascinating, peaceful, flowing, restful—that it needn't be highly organized or competitive. Perhaps you have forgotten the natural play of your childhood, when you could lose yourself in exploring rocks, making a fantasy realm out of a chair and a bedsheet, or singing for your own amusement.

It is easy to get caught up in the frenzy of filling every minute of your working hours with meaningful business. But this becomes a self-defeating strategy when it flows into your leisure time as well. The fear of "wasting" time has become an obsession for many, so they end up once again on a fast track of play.

"Chill out," teenagers suggest. "Relax, baby." "Don't have a cow," says cartoon character Bart Simpson. And these admonitions are important to keep in mind as you approach the subject of play. Please don't use any of the ideas here to burden yourself with any more de-

. . . .

Imagine the world without pleasure. Life would
appear colorless and humorless, a baby's smile
would go unappreciated. Foods would be tasteless.
The genius of a Bach concerto would fall on deaf
ears. Feelings like joy, thrills, delights, ecstasy,
elation, and happiness would disappear.
The company of others would bring no comfort or joy.
The touch of a mother would no longer soothe, and a
lover could not arouse. Interest in sex and procreation
would dry up. The next generation would await unborn.

—ORNSTEIN and SOBEL, *Healthy Pleasures*

. . . .

mands on your time and energy. Perhaps it's time to just do nothing for some part of each day, simply because it's good for your health. Slowing down long enough to receive the simple pleasures that are all around you is one of the most effective ways to deepen your enjoyment of life and thereby enhance your overall health. (See Processes 3, 9, 11, 15, and 16 for additional ways to slow down and enjoy your life.)

What's Your Pleasure? . . . .

What does play mean to you? Is there enough fun in your life? Enough time for simply fooling around? You will find it easier to begin exploring this subject by making a list of things that *aren't* fun or playful or enjoyable for you. Things like skydiving (which others love!), or shopping for clothes, or jogging. You may even get a laugh or two out of making the list. Once that list is out of the way, you may be more inspired to make a list of what *is* fun for you. Like checking out garage sales, going out for breakfast with a friend, or taking a sauna.

Next, go through your second list and indicate the last time you can remember taking part in each of these activities. Is there one item on your list that you could do today? One that you will put on your schedule for this or next week? Many people also find it helpful to schedule in times for just doing nothing.

. . . .

We stake our lives on our purposeful programs and projects, our serious jobs and endeavors. But doesn't the really important part of our life unfold "after hours"— singing and dancing, music and painting, prayer and lovemaking, or just fooling around?

—FR. WILLIAM MCNAMARA

. . . .

Resources

Wellness Workbook, 148–64.

Cousins, N. *Anatomy of an Illness.* New York: W. W. Norton and Co. 1979.

Moody, R. *Laugh After Laugh: The Healing Power of Humor.* Jacksonville, FL: Headwaters Press, 1978.

Peter, L. J., and B. Dana, *The Laughter Prescription.* New York: Ballantine Books, 1982.

Part III

Taking Action

Your leisurely hike along the foothills now brings you to the base of the mountain. The path of ascent stretches before you, sometimes rocky, sometimes steep. In Part III you will encounter processes that demand more of a commitment, and the decision to make wellness a way of life rather than a hobby or weekend diversion. When you decide to alter your diet, for instance, results may not be immediately apparent. In fact, you may actually go through a period of feeling worse before you start to feel better, since your body will have to cope with the symptoms of withdrawal from sugar and other addictive substances. Thus, the need for commitment.

We suggest that you start with the processes that address your most pressing concern—nutrition, exercise, relationships, communication, etc.—and that you use the resources suggested at the end of each section to deepen your self-understanding. Work on one area alone for at least several weeks before moving on to another area. Refer back to the processes in Part I and Part II, especially those that will support you as your start your climb, that is, as you start taking action.

The processes in Part III include:
- aerobic exercise
- nutritional awareness and dietary change
- building friendships
- listening skills for improved communications
- commonsense safety measures
- assertiveness training
- creating a healthier work environment
- cleaning up your environment

Move for the Health of It—
Do Something Aerobic

· · · · ·

$\mathcal{E}$verything inside you is moving. The heart pumps, blood flows, lungs expand and contract, eyes roll, eardrums vibrate, atoms dance, neurons fire. Outside, you walk, you reach out and touch the world around you, you stretch yourself, you dance. Movement is a sign of life. Seriously inhibit the movement of limbs and organs, and you encourage illness. Stop motion altogether and you are dead. Allow yourself to move as fully as possible both within and without, and you realize wellness.

Since the Industrial Revolution, life has changed dramatically. People no longer chop wood and carry water. Earning a livelihood more likely involves sitting for long hours at a desk or in an automobile, or standing behind a counter or at an assembly line. With rare exception, people's needs to move vigorously are few. Cars, buses, trains, planes, telephones, computers, overnight letters, and fax machines do it for them.

· · · · · · ·

*The labor of the human body is rapidly being
engineered out of working life.*

—JOHN F. KENNEDY

· · · · · · ·

Is this country turning into a nation of overweight couch potatoes? Statistics indicate that the average eighth grader can't pass a minimal fitness test, and most people think nothing about driving their car to a destination a few blocks away instead of walking. Heart disease is the leading cause of death in the US—and lack of exercise is one of the primary risk factors in its development.

Without exercise at all, as happens when you are confined to bed due to illness or accident, the muscles lose 15 percent of their strength for every week of inactivity. So, if you lead a sedentary life, chances are that your muscles are weak and therefore more injury-prone. But the good news is that this strength can be regained and the heart can be reconditioned. The body is amazingly resilient. Even years of neglect can be compensated for by a regular program of aerobic physical exercise. And more people than ever are doing just that. Thirty million Americans are now running or participating in some form of regular exercise. How about you?

NOT JUST JOGGING

Aerobics is any system of conditioning exercises that increases heart and breathing rates for a sustained period and thus increases the flow of oxygen and blood to all parts of the body. To be effective, the exercise must raise the pulse rate to a certain level (see chart below) and keep it at that level for not less than 10 or 15 minutes. (Note: People who are not in condition will have to build up slowly to a sustained 10- or 15-minute exercise period.)

Aerobic conditioning benefits the body in many ways. There will be a decrease in intramuscular fat and an increase in lean muscle, leading to a firmer, stronger body. Aerobic exercise is known to improve circulation because a trained heart is a more efficient pump and therefore

Heart Rates: (Based on resting heart rates of 72 for males and 80 for females.)			
AGE	RECOMMENDED TRAINING RATE	AGE	RECOMMENDED TRAINING RATE
20	160	36	149
22	158	38	147
24	157	40	146
25	155	45	143
28	154	50	140
30	152	55	137
32	151	60	128
34	150	65 +	120

doesn't have to work as hard. This lowered heart rate preserves the heart and lessens its chance of fatiguing prematurely. Aerobics will improve absorption and utilization of food; provide overall increases in energy and stamina; encourage more restful sleep; and decrease dependence on addictive substances such as alcohol, drugs, and tobacco. Most exercisers report a decrease in nervous tension and depression. And it is now known that exercise also causes the release of certain brain chemicals (endorphins and enkephalins) that increase the overall sense of well-being.

If you are not in the habit of exercising regularly, you may hear the word "aerobics," and immediately see visions of thin, tight bodies in shimmering leotards, or think with dread about jogging or running. Don't be discouraged. A wellness approach to exercise is not that limited.

DESIGN YOUR OWN PROGRAM

Every body is different, and every psyche is different, too. If you are someone who has resisted exercise in the past but knows now that it's time for a change, it is especially important that you design a program you can live with and stay with—a gentle, step-by-step program that will appeal to your fun-loving inner child, or provide companionship or quiet time alone, depending on your own special needs. Jogging or running are definitely not the only ways to move the body. Consider these other forms of aerobic exercise:

- dancing of all kinds (even ballroom dancing can elevate the heart rate)
- swimming and other water programs, including aerobics for non-swimmers
- walking, walking, walking, walking, walking
- hiking and climbing
- bicycling
- skipping, jumping rope, or rebounding on a trampoline
- calisthenics and weight training
- rowing
- tennis and other ball sports

- use of indoor equipment like stationary bikes, treadmills, or rowing machines

- Choose one or more forms of aerobic exercise that you think you will enjoy and try them out. You know yourself which exercise form you are more likely to stay with. Avoid setting yourself up for failure and disappointment by forcing yourself to be brave or strong about your exercise. Taking a vigorous walk around your block every day is infinitely more beneficial than dreaming about doing a triathalon.

. . . .

But if the dance of the run isn't fun
then discover another dance
because without fun
the good of the run
is undone
and a suffering runner
always quits
sooner or later.

—FRED ROHE, *The Zen of Running*

. . . .

- Don't be in a hurry. It takes time to recondition the heart. Before starting a program, a physical exam and an EKG are recommended, especially if you are over 40. Make realistic goals for yourself and reward every effort. Promise yourself small, healthy treats for accomplishing, or even approximating, your goals.

- Regular exercise is imperative. Three times a week, your exercise should maintain the training pulse rate for at least 15 minutes (See chart.) Block out exercise time in your weekly calendar. Call a friend and plan to exercise together. Keep a daily log of your progress, etc. Do anything and everything that will keep you moving.

- Always start your exercise with stretching warm-ups, and complete it with a cooling-down period that also includes stretching.

- Avoid imitation. Treasure your own uniqueness, even if you are working with a professional coach. Learn from the pros but don't hold yourself back by comparing yourself with them. And deal cautiously with competition—even if it's with yourself. Let yourself lose, or win, graciously.

- Follow spontaneous impulses and use every means available to stay inspired. When the urge to move arises, seize it. Close the office door and jump rope, or hang up the phone and run around the house.

- Breathe. Inhale as your movements expand, exhale as they contract or move back to center. You are overexerting if you can't talk comfortably as you exercise, or if your heart rate is not back to 120, or less, 5 minutes after completing your exercise. Normal breathing should return within 10 minutes after exertion.

- If pain starts, stop. Honor the body's natural warning system, especially in the beginning stages. Danger signs after which you should stop exercising include faintness, dizziness, nausea, tightness or pain in the chest, severe shortness of breath, or loss of muscle control.

- Whatever you're doing—dance it. Practice moving from "the inside out," smoothly, as if you were dancing, and the sense of rightness and connectedness that follows will make exercising a pleasant experience. When exercising outdoors, dance with the earth as you move on it.

Two Exercise Breaks . . . .

I. Take a walk. Walk briskly for at least 10 to 15 minutes. Start out at the rate of approximately 3 miles per hour. Move your whole body. Don't be afraid to swing your arms as you walk, since this will create a massaging action on the lymph glands in your armpits and stimulate the natural detoxifying function of these glands. Enjoy looking around at your environment as you walk along. Listen to the birds and smell the flowers.

Build up the length of time you spend walking by increasing it by 5 minutes a week until you can easily do 2 miles in about 30 minutes (35 minutes for women, 28 minutes for men). What could be simpler as a way to start your aerobic conditioning than to do something you've been doing all your life? More people are turning to walking as their preferred form of exercise because it is so much easier on the legs than running or jogging, and because there is no need for special equipment except a comfortable pair of walking shoes.

II. Join the Dance. You may be surprised at how easy and joyful movement can be. The exercise that follows is designed to get you dancing in a way that is energizing and fun. Read the directions over once or twice before you begin so that you won't have to stop once the movement starts. Here's what to do:

1. Play a recording of a slow, gentle piece of music, or tune your radio to a classical or "easy listening" station. Then close your eyes and simply listen to the music for a few minutes. Breathe it in.

2. Begin to move by directing your attention to your right hand and starting to tap or stretch your fingers in any way that the music suggests. Allow the movement to extend itself, to encompass your wrist as well. Keep doing this simple movement for a little while. Then direct your attention to the left hand and do the same. Imagine that you are directing an orchestra, or splashing in water, or molding a piece of clay to represent what you are hearing. Play with it. Next, engage your right arm, and then your left, allowing yourself to move from shoulders to tips of fingers. How many different ways can you find to bend them, to position them, to move them in unison or in opposition?

3. Keep your arms and hands going, doing whatever they want to, as you give attention to your head. Let the music direct it. Conduct the symphony with a baton that extends from the center of your forehead, from the crown, from your chin.

4. Your upper body now wants to get into the act. Concentrate on your middle section. Allow yourself to bend and sway from the waist in any ways that feel good. Pretend that your whole body exists from waist to head—forget the rest. Let the hips and pelvis come along whenever you are ready for them. Careful here—they will want to take over.

5. Imagine yourself as a tree in the wind. Roots are firm. Only the branches and upper trunk sway. Be a fettered bird, wanting to escape, but restrained by a silver thread. Fantasize that you are a belly dancer, write your name with an imaginary pencil that extends from your left hip. Write "I love you" with the imaginary pencil on your right hip.

6. Unlock your knees and allow your legs to move without lifting your feet. Challenge yourself with how many ways you can direct them, ways that you have never tried before. Pretend that you are scientifically cataloguing all the possible combinations of movement that legs can make. Keep your feet still until you can't stand it a minute

longer. Go within yourself and take note of what your body feels like all over. Imagine your blood cells dancing, oxygen dancing, energy dancing.

7. Now let go completely and allow yourself to move totally—head, arms, belly, pelvis, legs, feet. Surprise!

Want another exercise? Try a different, perhaps more active, piece of music.

Resources

Wellness Workbook, 91–108.

Cooper, K. *The Aerobics Program for Total Well-Being.* New York: Bantam Books, 1982.

Rohe, F. *The Zen of Running.* Berkeley, CA: Random House/Bookworks, 1974.

Yanker, G. *Walking Medicine.* New York: McGraw Hill, 1990.

Develop Personal Nutritional Awareness

· · · · ·

$\mathcal{F}$ood and nutrition are enormously popular subjects today. Food companies are climbing on the bandwagon, offering products that are vitamin enriched, low in salt, high in fiber, or caffeine- or cholesterol-free. People are preoccupied with cutting down on fat and cholesterol. At the same time they are inclined, because of their high-speed life-styles, to eat more fast foods, which are notoriously high in both. For many people, confusion has increased with the numerous choices offered and the growing body of nutritional information. Since even the experts often disagree among themselves, it's no wonder that nutrition has become a subject that is almost as controversial as religion or politics.

In the 1960s, the pioneering work of Roger J. Williams, PhD, introduced the concept of biochemical individuality—the understanding that each person has unique biochemical needs that can only be met by a specific balance of nutrients that fills those needs. His work ushered in the era of individual nutritional analysis, the metabolic profile, the personalized health plan, and the specially designed diet. While such workups may be valuable, unless they rest on a foundation of self-understanding, they become one more way of putting your well-being in the control of others. The point is that you need to develop awareness of your own nutritional needs and understand your own relationship to foods. Then you can become a partner with the experts, using the information they supply to supplement what you know about yourself. Then you can decide what makes nutritional sense for you.

Process 6 spoke generally of tuning in to your body's feedback system, of listening to and inhabiting your body. What follows builds on these concepts, applying this awareness specifically to food and eating habits. We suggest that you review Process 6 before proceeding.

As far as food is concerned, developing awareness of your body means that you observe—with honesty, sensitivity, and thoroughness—

what types and quantities of food and what eating environments support your overall well-being, and what foods or environments don't. For instance, when food is eaten so quickly that you don't have time to taste it, or when it is used to soothe emotional pain, or when you get in the habit of overeating, you soon lose awareness of what food is doing for you. As you sharpen your ability to "hear" what your body is telling you about its relationship to food, you reinforce the conscious lifestyle that you have chosen to live. This type of awareness is an effective way of breaking the dieting habit forever. Instead of waging war with the body, you form an alliance with it, feeding it what it really wants and needs to support you.

TAKING STOCK

1. Find out what you are eating, when, and how the food makes you feel by keeping a nutritional journal for a week or more. Record anything that you learn about your relationship to food and use the finding in your journal, eventually, to design a simpler and healthier diet for yourself. (See sample journal on p.79.)

2. Pause for a moment and become aware of how hungry your body feels. Ask yourself, on a scale of 1 to 10, where 1 = fainting from hunger and 10 = overstuffed, just how hungry you are now. Do this several times during the day to heighten your self-awareness and get in the habit of eating only when your awareness score is 5 or less. Learn to distinguish between *stomach hunger* and *mouth hunger*. Mouth hunger is usually experienced in the jaws, tongue, teeth, and gums, which want to chew on or be stimulated by something, or in a salivary reaction prompted by the sight of food or such cues as a restaurant sign or the noon whistle. Mouth hunger is often an indication of the need for attention, affection, pain relief, or security of some sort.

3. Observe bodily signs that indicate imbalances in your diet. Look at your tongue, for instance. If it is frequently discolored or coated, or if you consistently have bad breath or a sour taste in your mouth, realize that these are important signs of the need for a change. The health of your gums and teeth are indicators of both good dental care and a healthy diet. Teeth can become discolored from caffeine and nicotine, and eating foods with lots of sugar can contribute to the development of cavities. Fingernails that split may mean that your

body is not assimilating protein properly. "Read" your bowel movements for signs of a poor diet. If stools are hard to pass and dark, and sink rather than float, dietary change is indicated. Many processed foods, like white flour products, are slow to move through the intestines. Eating foods with a high fiber content, adding a moderate amount of oil (like olive or canola) to the diet, and drinking lots of water will speed intestinal transit time, lowering your risk of colon or intestinal cancer and improving your health in general.

A Nutrition Journal

A nutrition journal can be used as:
- your personal record of the ways your body responds to the foods you eat

- a balance sheet to observe the kinds of raw materials/fuels with which you supply your body

- a place to keep special recipes

- a diet notebook for weight gain/loss

- a record of emotions felt, resolutions, etc.

For example:
Subject Under Consideration: Breakfast

Day/Time
Monday 3/22 9:00 AM

Breakfast Foods:
2 eggs, bacon—2 strips, toast—2 pieces, butter and jam
coffee—2 cups

Immediate Effects/Later Effects
Left the table feeling stuffed. Too much food.
Generally good day. Not hungry until 3:00 PM

Reflections:

Resolutions:

---

4. Consider headaches as loud and clear messages that something about the organism is amiss. Frequently they are indicative of stress, but they are also associated with a host of dietary problems, such as excessive alcohol consumption and blood sugar imbalances.

5. Frequent indigestion? Listening to your body means carefully noting how you feel after eating certain foods. *Indigestion is not normal.* If you get up from the table or wake up in the morning feeling nauseated, bloated, heavy, achy, etc., it's time for a change of menu.

6. Difficulty in sleeping? Try to recall what food and drink you consumed in the hours before retiring. Many people find that heavy foods, caffeine drinks, or chocolate and other sweets interfere with their ability to fall asleep quickly and stay asleep.

THEN WHAT?

Experiment with certain foods and certain ways of eating. Allow enough time in each experiment to really experience the effects. Add a food or stop eating a particular food for a while. Try eating your heaviest meal in the middle of the day, for instance, or abstaining from food for three to four hours before retiring.

Educate yourself about nutrition. Read. Inquire of your health professionals or those who exemplify healthiness for you. Go on to Process 17.

Resources

Wellness Workbook, 64–90.

Bland, J. *Your Health Under Siege: Using Nutrition to Fight Back.* New York: Penguin Books, 1984.

Saltoon, D. *The Common Book of Consciousness: How to Take Charge of Your Lifestyle through Diet, Exercise and Meditation.* Berkeley, CA: Celestial Arts Publishing, 1991.

Williams, R. *Biochemical Individuality.* Austin, TX: University of Texas Press, 1969.

——— . *Nutrition Against Disease.* New York: Bantam Books, 1978.

Ten Basics about Food

· · · · ·

$\mathcal{T}$his book doesn't prescribe a single system that everyone can or should follow. That would undermine the concept of self-trust that is its underlying premise. However, some consideration of the components of sound nutritional practice is needed if you are to develop a diet that will truly support your well-being. Although a mass of confusing data surrounds this subject, certain recommendations are almost universally accepted, and these warrant your attention. The guidelines originally offered in 1977 by the McGovern Committee on Nutrition and Human Needs have stood the test of time and represent a balanced approach. They are presented here, together with a few additional suggestions of our own, for your consideration.

· · · · · · ·

Simple diets have nourished
humans for millions of years.
Why stop now?

—J.W.T.

· · · · · · ·

Ten Nutrition Basics:

1. Increase your consumption of fruits, vegetables, and whole grains. These foods contain vitamins and minerals in their natural form as well as fiber, which has been shown to markedly reduce the risk of bowel cancer and other diseases of the intestines. The lower on the food chain your diet is, and the simpler, the healthier you will be.

2. Decrease consumption of highly processed foods, especially those that contain additives and preservatives. These foods have less nutritional value because many desirable components have been pro-

cessed out of them, decreasing their "life force" or vitality. These same foods are then "enriched" and "preserved" with additives. Over time, the extra work of dealing with these additives takes a cumulative toll on your liver, which must break down, detoxify, or store the unusable substances found in processed foods.

3. Decrease your consumption of red meat. Red meat is unnecessary in a carefully chosen human diet. Diets high in red meat are linked to heart disease and bowel cancer.

4. Reduce overall consumption of fats, particularly animal fats. A high intake of fats is implicated in heart disease, cancer, and obesity.

5. Reduce consumption of foods containing high amounts of cholesterol. A high intake of cholesterol is also implicated in heart disease and cancer.

6. Decrease consumption of sugar and foods high in added sugar. Eliminating or substantially reducing the use of processed sweets may not be easy since sugar does provide a quick, short-lived burst of energy which you may have come to rely on. Sugar stresses both the liver and pancreas as they work to counterbalance the effects of the sugar rush. Decreasing your intake of sugar will give your body a chance to rest from such chronic overstress. It will increase the efficiency of all your digestive organs, resulting in better physical energy in the long run. Many people who stop the processed-sugar habit find that they have significantly fewer mood swings, headaches, and erratic food cravings. Furthermore, the calories obtained from junk foods create a substitution effect and decrease your appetite for the foods that would give you the nutrients you need.

7. Use less salt. The daily requirement of salt in the diet is only about one-half gram (about three shakes of salt shaker) and most likely the unsalted foods you eat contain more than that. The daily salt consumption in the US ranges from 6 to 18 grams. Salt has been found to increase blood pressure and hypertension, and some reports link high salt intake with changes in levels of gastric acid secretion, stomach cancer, and cerebrovascular disease. Salt crystals can accumulate in the kidneys, leading to pain and the formation of kidney stones.

8. Reduce or completely eliminate the use of caffeine. Caffeine continually overstimulates the adrenal glands, causing the secretion of

adrenaline into your bloodstream. This is why you feel such a rush from caffeine products. The liver must overcompensate to keep the caffeine from affecting the heart, and overall, this depletes your energy. When energy flags, many people simply ingest more caffeine. This erratic pattern is highly stressful on your liver and other organs. Caffeine is clearly an addictive substance, as anyone who has tried to withdraw from it knows.

9. Drink lots of pure water—ideally eight glasses a day. Most people are chronically dehydrated and don't realize it (see Process 12). If you are not sure that your tap water is pure, have it tested.

10. Exercise daily to encourage maximum utilization of the foods you are eating. If possible, exercise outdoors but away from running automobiles and other sources of air pollution.

An Exercise in Good Nutrition . . . .

Think about your food consumption over the past two or three days. Does it reflect, essentially, the recommendations listed above? Which guidelines do you currently adhere to regularly?

Which ones are more difficult for you to implement in your daily diet?

Choose one or two of the 10 basics above that you will implement over the course of the next few weeks. Don't burden yourself with trying to change everything at once. Write a contract with yourself stating what you will do, how long you will do it, and what you will move on to next. For instance: "From now until the end of the month I will eat at least one fresh fruit each day, and I will cut down on my use of table salt. Next month I will work on eating at least one serving of raw or lightly steamed vegetables each day."

My contract with myself:

You may find it helpful to tape this contract onto the refrigerator, or share this exercise with a friend, someone who will remind you of your contract and encourage you to keep it. Invite your friend to do the same.

Resources

Wellness Workbook, 64–90.

Natow, A., and Heslin, J. *Nutrition for the Prime of Your Life.* New York: McGraw-Hill, 1983.

Robertson, L., Flinders, C., and Godfrey, B. *Laurel's Kitchen: A Handbook for Vegetarian Cooking and Nutrition.* Berkeley, CA: Ten Speed Press, 1987.

Urs Koch, M. *Laugh with Health.* New York: Holt, Rinehart and Winston, 1981.

··········· ·PROCESS **18**···

Prevent Accidents

· · · · ·

Commonsense safety is easily overlooked as an integral part of a program of personal wellness. A person may exercise extreme caution about diet, yet be quite lax in attending to accident prevention.

Most accidents—both in the home and on the road—are easily preventable. No training is needed to put on a seat belt in the car or to buckle up children, but these simple gestures can save lives and dramatically decrease the chances of severe injury. It only takes a minute to ask your doctor or pharmacist to check your prescription and over-the-counter medications for possible adverse drug interactions. Over half of all prescriptions dispensed annually are taken incorrectly, and drug errors account for increasing numbers of deaths in hospitals and nursing homes.

You already know most of what is needed to prevent accidents, since most of it is basic, common sense. Yet the complications and pressures of modern life may cause you to put these safety precautions low on your list of priorities. The memory jogger below is designed to encourage you to take action where it is needed.

A Safety Survey . . . .

Jot down here what you already know about each of the items listed below, or go over this list with your spouse, your children, or a friend, and use it as a basis for discussion.

What I know about safety and wellness with regard to:

home fire extinguishers

icy sidewalks and steps

use and maintenance of stairs and handrails

slippery floors and movable area rugs

wet, slippery surfaces, especially bathtubs

children's access to prescription or over-the-counter drugs

out-of-date prescriptions or over-the-counter drugs

seat belts and air bags

automobile tires, wiper blades, and antilock brakes

car safety seats for children

the speed limit

driving or operating machinery under the influence of alcohol or drugs

escape plans in case of fire both at home and away

overloaded, improperly fused electrial outlets

frayed electrical wires

use of electrical equipment near water

space heaters

storing cleaning products, medicines, and poisons in homes where children live or visit using household cleaning products and pesticides that contain toxic substances

emergency phone numbers

accessibility of first-aid supplies

first-aid skills for choking, burns, shock, etc.

protection from high-volume sound

safe disposal of paints, paint thinners, gasoline, oil

children's toys

This list is not comprehensive. It is meant as a place to start. We suggest that you add to it by taking a slow walk through and around your home, looking for safety hazards. Make notes on what you know needs to be done. Check off a few items that you need to do something about as soon as possible. Prioritize your checked items. Take a calendar and assign, in order of priority, one item to next week, and one or more items to each month for the remainder of the year and into next year if necessary.

If you need more information about any of the items, your public library is an excellent place to start. Consult the front pages of your phone book, which, in most areas, has a survival guide and emergency numbers. Call your local Red Cross for information about safety training.

Resources

Wellness Workbook, "Wellness Index Questionnaire," section 1.

Dadd, D. *The Non-Toxic Home: Protecting Yourself and Your Family from Everyday Toxics and Health Hazards.* Los Angeles, CA: J. P. Tarcher, 1986.

Nader, R. *The Home Book.* (Available from P.O. Box 19367, Washington, DC 20036.)

Keep Friendship Alive

The opposite of love is not hate, but indifference.
—ANONYMOUS

· · · · ·

*P*eople need people. And often they don't realize how great their need is until some moment of great joy or deep sorrow. At some point in your life you've probably experienced this yourself—wanting to share some great news with a friend or, perhaps during hard times, needing care and support from others.

Less obvious is the need for strong positive relationships on a day-to-day basis. Just as children need to be physically touched, stroked, and held in order to develop normally, all people need emotional stroking for a healthy, well-balanced life. A "stroke," in the language of Trans-actional Analysis (TA), is any form of stimulation or recognition that arouses feelings. Strokes may be positive, such as smiles, hugs, and loving words, or negative, like brush-offs, cold stares, slaps, or repri-mands. Whether they are positive or negative, strokes confirm that you exist and that you matter, and this validation is essential to healthy human survival.

The alarming thing to realize is that if people don't get their strokes in life-affirming ways, they will seek them out in death-promoting ways rather than suffer the condition of being a nonentity. Illnesses of body, mind, and spirit are used by many people, both consciously and uncon-sciously, to get strokes, since they provide attention, touching, stimu-lation, and something to do.

One of the healthiest things you can do for yourself is to cultivate vibrant friendships—the kind that will supply you with the genuine stroking everyone needs, friendships in which you can dare to reveal your feelings, dare to act spontaneously, dare to care, to touch, to serve. Stimulating and supportive relationships with other human beings are tremendous blessings—to the body, the mind, and the spirit.

A 20-year survey of adults in the US indicated that, regardless of health problems, people who participated in formal social networks of some type outlived those who didn't. An affiliation with a social network was found to be the strongest predictor of longevity, even above age, sex, or health. "When people are counting on you, you have a reason to get up in the morning," one researcher said. A 1984 Ohio State University study found that medical students with the highest loneliness scores and highest stress had depressed immune system functioning. In other words, they were more susceptible to disease.

KEEPING A RELATIONSHIP VIBRANT

Rich human relationships aren't sustained by accident, or made once and for all. A good marriage lasts because it is renewed day after day after day. Healthy relationships of all kinds will last and deepen if, like other growing things, they are watered and fed, and even pruned on a regular basis. Making the sustenance and maintenance of friendships a part of everyday life is an invaluable enhancement of wellness.

Following are some suggestions from long-term friends and married partners for simple things you can do to nourish relationships that are important to you and to guarantee a stroke-rich environment for yourself.

- **Respect the other,** despite disagreement over issues. Approach your mate or your friend with the same deference that you would pay to some hero or heroine—a great person you admire. Honor the differences between you and avoid trying to control the other, even subtly, to suit your ideas of who they are or how they should be. Encourage conversation that allows you each to share your goodness of spirit.

- **Be brand-new,** and allow your friends and partners to be brand-new, too. Recognize another human being as a profound mystery that will never be "solved." When you give up presuppositions about the way someone has "always been" you literally give the other the green light to change and grow. If you keep remembering to be new, you are more likely to continue the courtship—dress for dinner, or bring flowers, or listen to the other's stories—with the same exhilaration and respect that you had when you first met.

- **Give attention to small gestures** that will provide pleasure or happiness to your friend or partner. A hot cup of tea brought to the bed

87

in the morning, the remembrance of the other with a small gift or a card—these are the little touches that build great friendships.

- **Take risks and continue to share something new.** Keep growing in new ways yourself. Taking risks may be as simple as taking a seminar or other educational course, reading books in areas that you generally don't explore, or travelling. Money needn't be an obstacle to experimentation and surprise. Honor your own dreams and keep working for them. That builds your self-esteem and invites your friends and partners to do the same.

- **Retain some rituals.** Celebrate holidays or anniversaries of important occasions, or share your spiritual or religious practices with your friends and family. Honor your traditions and your roots.

- **Pray for each other.** Whatever form prayer takes in your life—a traditional religious form or a simple positive mental remembrance—it is a significant way to build your connections beyond mere physical contact.

- **Put attention into honest communication,** especially through empathic listening. (See Process 20 for help in this area.) Set aside times in which you will periodically clear the air of any questions or resentments that may have been building between you. Read a book together about how to improve communications, or take a class or seminar on the subject. Give yourself permission to say no as well as yes to your friend, and you will be doing your friend a great favor in the long run.

Right Now: Before reading any more in this book or starting another project, take five minutes to write a two- or three-line note of appreciation or thanks to someone you care about. Send it out in the next mail.

Resources

Wellness Workbook, 185–95.

Betcher, W. *Intimate Play: Creating Romance in Everyday Life.* New York: Penguin Books, 1988.

Energize Your Communication— Become a Genuine Listener

· · · · ·

*S*ince almost half the time you spend in communication is spent in listening, you should be an expert at it by now. If you are, though, you are the rare exception. Most people listen passively, planning what they are going to say next, or they listen partially, jumping on the first few words and extrapolating the rest. It is no wonder that communication often lacks energy and leaves people feeling drained, bored, joyless, angry, depressed, or helpless. In many conversations there is little actual communication and poor listening is usually at the root of the problem.

Dynamic listening is more than simply hearing. And it is easy to confuse the two. Think about this distinction in the realm of music. You probably hear music of some sort almost every day—as background to a TV show or in the supermarket. Even if you are not consciously aware of hearing it, this music creates a mood. Rarely will you attend to the lyrics or dance to the rhythm of this kind of music. Now contrast this with your behavior at a concert, a symphony, or a dance. In these circumstances, your body is turned in the direction of the band or orchestra. You experience an emotional rush, perhaps, as you allow the music in. You may involve your body with it, starting to sway or hum along, or to clap in time. When it ends, you will applaud or stand up and shout. Now you are really listening dynamically.

Imagine giving that kind of attention to another human being—involving yourself actively in what they are saying. That's what it means to *listen* rather than merely to *hear*. Active listening forms the basis of strong interpersonal relationships. It encourages interaction with the other, rather than the assumption of a passive role like the one people usually take with doctors, teachers, and other experts. It allows you to step inside the other person's shoes and to see, hear, and feel the world from their perspective. With that advantage, miracles can happen between you and others.

. . . .

*I believe the greatest gift I can conceive of having
from anyone is to be seen by them, heard by them,
to be understood and touched by them. The greatest
gift I can give is to see, hear, understand and to
touch another person. When this is done I feel
contact has been made.*

—VIRGINIA SATIR

. . . .

Good listeners are made, not born. They are made by their willingness to observe the volumes that are spoken between the lines in ordinary conversation. Good listeners, for instance, "hear" a clenched fist, or a softened voice, or a look in the eye as much as they hear the words of the other. A good listener is patient and nonjudgmental. A good listener gives room to other people's views without immediately trying to correct them or help them. A good listener assumes that the one speaking is *the expert* about themselves, and essentially strives to become a witness to a process of self-discovery on the part of the speaker. A good listener isn't satisfied with partial data and doesn't presume to know what the other person means. A good listener will ask questions to clarify meaning and will often paraphrase what was heard to see if it was understood. A good listener is an active presence. A good listener will look at you, smile, nod the head, or give other appropriate forms of nonverbal feedback. (Too much of this, however, can be a sign of trying to please without really listening.) A good listener can be a very good friend.

. . . .

*When you listen to me without interruption or
anything that feels like a judgement, you
allow me the time and space to get more in
touch with the many facets of me.
Thank you for never playing with my words,
getting a laugh or recognition at my expense.
When you allow me to revise or restructure what I
have said, I feel that you are truly committed
to understanding me and what I'm about.
Thank you for not feeling that you necessarily
have to do something about what I share.*

When you listen, I feel that you are listening
not only to my words but the feelings
 behind them.
Bless you for being you and thereby assisting me
 in my journey.

—BENNETT KILPACK

· · · · · · ·

BARRIERS TO GOOD LISTENING

The first step in any process of change is to become aware of what you are doing at present. You are probably not aware of the barriers you habitually put up to block good communication. Look over the list below and identify any that you use.

Evaluating and judging. Are you so busy criticizing what the other is saying that you don't hear them? There is nothing wrong with using discrimination, but it is more helpful to defer judgement until you fully understand what the other person is talking about.

Interrupting. When you don't allow the other person to complete a thought, you are not listening. Many people will interrupt because they are impatient. If you find yourself losing the train of the conversation because the other is talking excessively, ask for a summary and then continue to listen.

Jumping to conclusions. It is easy to mentally fill in the details of what another person is saying and then to assume you have understood them. People often take everything they hear personally—one of the main reasons for the misunderstandings that lead to breakdowns in relationships. You can remedy that tendency by checking out your assumptions first.

Selective listening. People tend to hear what they expect to hear, need to hear, or want to hear and block out the rest. For example, if you have been feeling a lack of confidence in yourself lately, you might hear everything that is said to you through a filter of "I'm no good." Or you might tune out everything that is critical, unpleasant, or negative because it is too threatening to hear right now. Keep in mind that everybody uses some form of selective listening. Get to know your own kind and observe your tendency to block listening with it.

Advising. You may think that you have to answer every question asked and solve every problem. Not true. The other may be simply thinking aloud, asking rhetorical questions, or just looking for a supportive presence. In fact, as you share your advice, you may actually be disregarding what the other is saying. Let others specifically ask for help or advice. Otherwise, just listen and "be there." One valuable way to encourage people to solve their own problems is to ask how they would advise a friend with a similar problem.

Lack of attention. Do you let your mind wander frequently in conversations, giving in to other external noises and distractions or to your own daydreams or plans? Often it is helpful to be up front about it—admit your temporary lack of attention to the person speaking; explain that you are sleepy, anxious, or whatever. If boredom is the problem though, remember that the more *involved* you become in the conversation the less boring it may be. Ask questions. Ask for examples. Summarize what you hear the other person saying. If all else fails tell the other person honestly that you need to leave or get back to work, etc. Good listening need not be a matter of silent endurance. Good listening is an active process.

TOWARDS DYNAMIC LISTENING

Consider which of the listening blocks cited above are yours. When do you most frequently use them? With whom? Why? Choose one block at which you would like to chip away. Who would you like to practice better listening with? Under what circumstances? Determine to watch yourself throughout your next interaction with that person, noticing how easily you fall into your habitual patterns of passivity or non-listening and/or how well you implement your new active listening behavior. Make a tally sheet for yourself of how many times in that conversation you "blocked" the communications; how many times you broke through the block with active listening. Write about your experience to help clarify it for yourself.

Remember, you cannot change the other person, but the quality of your relationship can be improved if you start to practice active listening.

Resources

Wellness Workbook, 165–84.

McKay, M., Davis, M., and Fanning, P. *Messages.* Oakland, CA: New Harbinger Publications, 1983.

Satir, V. *Making Contact.* Berkeley, CA: Celestial Arts, 1976.

Just Say No!

· · · · ·

$\mathcal{F}$amily therapist Virginia Satir used to wear a medallion around her neck. The word *yes* was emblazoned on one side of the medallion, and on the other side, the word *no*. She often said that one of her primary tasks was to help her clients learn simple assertiveness—to say yes when they meant yes, and no when they meant no.

Recently the need for assertiveness has been emphasized by those who work within the growing field of addiction "recovery"—in particular the recovery from codependence, which Virginia Satir estimated was present in over 90 percent of the US population. "The disease of lost selfhood," as author Charles Whitfield, MD, calls it, codependence is probably at the root of all other addictions. It results from focusing too much on what is outside of yourself and thereby depending on others to define what you think, how you feel, and what you do.

THE HIGH COST OF YES

While an attitude of openness to life is definitely health-promoting, saying yes to life means saying no a good deal of the time, too. People who are afraid of disapproval from others will say yes regardless of their true feelings, so as not to rock the boat. The question can range from the trivial ("Would you like a cup of coffee?") to the serious ("Can I stay at your apartment for a few weeks?"). When it comes to dealing with doctors or other caregivers, it is easy to fall into the trap of being the passive patient, afraid to say no to a suggested procedure, for instance, even though you may feel very ambivalent about it.

You will probably pay a high price for such a lack of assertiveness, in your personal relationships and in your dealings with professionals. Here's why:

It's stressful. Holding in feelings of anger or frustration while smiling and saying yes is a source of unnecessary tension, and if you do this continually it may erupt in physical symptoms or emotional confusion and instability.

It's confusing. Other people will "read" the true message in your body language, tone of voice, or energy level. They will be unsure of what you are really saying and will question your trustworthiness.

It's undermining of yourself. You erode your own self-esteem when you deny that you have the right to speak the truth as you see it. By saying yes when you mean no you give up your vote over what goes on in your own life. The more you deny yourself this right, the more you may feed feelings of low self-worth and set in motion the cycle of dishonesty/guilt/self-hatred/depression.

It's disempowering to others. When you assume that other people will be upset or fall apart because you say no, you are assuming they do not have the strength to hold on to their own convictions. Genuine friendship or colleagueship cannot grow from such a weak foundation. Loneliness is often the result.

Learning to Say No . . . .

Admittedly, saying no is not easy if a lifetime of yes has preceded it. You may find that you are suddenly less popular with certain people (especially those who are afraid to think for themselves). To practice saying no, you may want to start with matters of small consequence and work up to the bigger ones. Here are a variety of approaches:

- Practice on yourself. Stand in front of a mirror and practice saying no in a variety of ways. Experiment with different phrases that feel natural to you: "No thank you, but thanks for asking." "Doing that would require more (time, work, money) than I'm willing to spend right now." "I've decided to cut back on my involvements to put more time into my (home life, school work, relationship with my spouse, etc.)."

- Write out, in simple sentences, the clear "no" message that you may be afraid to deliver. Use this script when you need to call someone to say no or practice it before meeting someone in person. "I know that you need help on this project, and it was great to work on it with you last year, but I have other priorities at this time that require my attention, so I will be unable to assist you. Good luck in getting the volunteers you need, and please call me again for next year." Avoid apologizing. Practice your script until it sounds natural to you. The more you assert yourself in this way, the easier it will become.

- Examine the ways in which you currently spend your time and energy, including your diet and exercise programs. Determine which activities no longer support your well-being. Make a list of *no mores* and post it where you will see it often. Check off one or two of the ones you could most easily drop and plan to get at this right away. Think back to the last time you wanted to say no but didn't. Recall, with as much detail as you can, your feelings about that situation. Forgive yourself for your lack of honesty, if that was the case. Decide whether you want to, if you can, remedy that situation by saying no now. In any case, reaffirm your intention to say no—as appropriate—in the future.

- Read over the Assertive Bill of Rights below. Use it often to encourage yourself to say no or yes as necessary.

Assertive Bill of Rights

I have the right to. . .

- be responsible for my own life

- support others being responsible for themselves

- create conscious interdependence in my life (we're all here together)

- accept and respect myself and others

- feel happy, satisfied, and to allow inner peace

- take good care of my whole being: my body, my mind, and my spirit

- be imperfect, and to forgive myself and others for our mistakes

- be aware of and fulfill my own needs (and to support others doing so also)

- have dreams, goals, and ideals—and to bring them into reality

- have and express all my emotions, without indulgence

- tell others how I want to be treated

- allow people to help me even if I'm feeling guilty, unworthy, or dependent

- set my own priorities for the use of time, money, space, and energy

- get what I pay for

- get paid what I deserve

- have healthy, life-enhancing relationships

- change, emerge, expand in new directions

- free myself from guilt and worry, and trust the goodness of myself

- work together with others to resolve conflict and build a world beyond war

—RUTH SHARON,
Conflict: A Way to Peace:
The AFDA Training Manual

Resources

Wellness Workbook, 165–84.

Alberti, R., and Emmons, M. *Your Perfect Right.* San Luis Obispo, CA: Impact Publishers, 1970.

Beattie, M. *Codependent No More.* New York: Harper and Row, 1987.

Fensterheim, H. and Baer, J. *Don't Say Yes When You Want to Say No.* New York: Dell, 1975.

Satir, V. *Peoplemaking.* Palo Alto, CA: Science and Behavior Books, 1988.

Sharon, R. *Conflict: A Way to Peace: The AFDA Training Manual.* Englewood, CO.

Work Well

You work that you may keep pace with the earth
and the soul of the earth.
—KAHLIL GIBRAN

· · · · ·

$\mathcal{T}$hese words of the poet came from an earlier time when people worked more directly to maintain their own survival—growing food, clearing the land, and building their own homes with tools of their own fabrication. But the principle still applies. There is an inherent value in sharing in the work of the world and doing one's part. In this sense there is no job that is ignoble.

But people tend to lose sight of the value of their work, to get so caught up in the details that they forget what they are doing or why they are doing it. Complaints are rife: too much pressure, too boring, the boss is impossible. Whatever the problem, the outcome is the same—job dissatisfaction leading to complete burnout—the feeling that you can't face another day on the job.

Most people spend a third or more of their lives in the workplace. It is very important, then, that work supports well-being in all ways— physically, emotionally, relationally, intellectually, etc. The body can put up with abuse in the short run, but over years those abuses will take their toll.

A Few Steps towards Healthier Work · · · · · · · · · · · ·

There are many ways to practice initiative and self-responsibility in the workplace without having to quit your job. It is possible to make changes in your relationship to your job so that it will satisfy you more deeply.

1. First, assess your relationship to your job in the light of the factors below.

- You like what you do even if you don't like all of the details of your job. Your job provides you with the opportunity to take on tasks, accomplish them, and feel good about yourself and about what you have created or produced.

- You have a sense of purpose in what you do. In other words, you have made the job important by the way in which you define or view it. You appreciate yourself for working to support yourself and your family, even if your job is not ideal.

- You can distinguish between the job you do and who you are. You know that even if you are unable to work or are unemployed, you are still a worthwhile human being.

- You spend time cultivating other interests and other aspects of yourself that your job doesn't include. You continue to learn, to stretch, to grow, and, especially, to take small risks as ways to keep yourself flexible in body, mind, and soul.

- You practice self-responsibility, safety, stress reduction, and honest communication as much as possible. You stand up as a person of clear integrity within your work environment.

- You feel good when you get up in the morning to go to work. You experience general good health and rarely find it necessary to take a sick leave to cope with the job.

- Your work is appreciated and encouraged by your spouse and children. It allows you to spend the quality time that you desire with your family.

2. Tell yourself the truth about your job and how it supports your well-being. Take a good long look at your job situation, as well as the physical conditions under which you work. Make it a thorough look.

   a. Imagine that you are a journalist doing a story on the healthiness of your workplace. Start making a list. Even though you may feel sure many things cannot be changed, list them anyway. Here are a few things to consider:

      - sufficiency and type of lighting

      - quality of the air that circulates in your workplace

- access to the natural environment

  —do you have a window in your area?

  —can plants grow there?

- colors on walls

- noise levels—of machinery or other workers

- interruptions by the telephone

- traffic patterns in your space

- design and placement of furniture

Review your list and ask yourself if these things serve your work and help you to work more efficiently and pleasantly, or if they undermine your health and your work.

b. Now examine the pace of work. Does your job allow for periodic stretches? Do you have to spend hours sitting, or do you have the opportunity to get up and walk around? (Many people may just settle for the inevitability of this instead of initiating something to change it.) Who sets deadlines? Are they generally realistic? Are you expected to work overtime regularly or take work home on weekends?

c. Look at the cultural norms in your office or work group. Is smoking or drinking encouraged? Are heavy lunches of high-fat food the usual fare? Is coffee the beverage that fuels the work? Do people support one another in exercise or working out in some way? Do you?

d. There may be some difficult people with whom it is necessary to interact. Are you able to maintain your sense of self-worth despite the activities of others? If not, what internal messages do you give yourself when you leave these people? Are you highly self-critical, defensive, upset? What do you and your co-workers talk about when you are not working? Do these conversations create momentum for creative action and uplift or stimulate you, or are they full of gossip and do they generally depress, drain, and bore you?

3. That's a lot of investigating. Maybe you've opened up a few cans of worms for yourself that you didn't want to touch. Summarize what you've discovered for yourself in some way. Write a letter to yourself in which you describe your current job situation in terms of health.

Or give yourself a job-health quotient by assigning yourself a score between 1 and 100, where 100 indicates an ideal, high-health work environment, and 1 means a work situation that is about to kill you.

4. No matter how bad the situation may seem, realize that when you give up your voice in your own life, you become the victim of circumstances, and then you are lost. If you maintain a sense of being in charge of your own life, you become an active participant. You do this by initiating changes, however small. Many times a small change is *all* it takes. (See Processes 3, 9, and 10 for breathing, stretching, and loosening up exercises that can be done at the workplace.)

Make a distinction here—there are two levels at which you can make changes. The first is at the level of behavior—here you will actually do something, or not do something, to effect a change in your environment. For years Regina adjusted her chair to suit the height of her word processor screen, but found that her legs were always cramped. Recently she decided to make her working environment healthier, so she put the screen on a stand that raised it by eight inches. Now her chair can stay higher, giving more room to her legs. Her neck doesn't have to be bent all day long, and she has discovered that the change has relieved some of her low-back pain. Other small changes at this level can include negotiation with management for a healthier environment or a change of schedules to allow for flextime. You could also confer with your co-workers to bring about some changes. This is more valuable than trying to be a lone crusader.

The second level of change is attitudinal change. Here you work within yourself, changing your perception, or your degree of attachment, or your sense of purpose and intention with regard to your job. The proverbial cup appears half empty or half full depending upon the attitude of the observer. It is up to you to define how your job gives meaning to your life and what overall purpose it serves. Meanings are in people, not in things. Recall Gibran's words and choose the meaning your work has for the soul of the earth. Remember, it is not always possible to change what is, but it is always possible to change your relationship to it. The books listed in the following resource section will assist you in making this reorientation.

You may decide that the only solution to your problem is a job change. This is not something to be done hastily, even if it is economically feasible. So take time to review Processes 1 and 2 on goal setting. Then, make a three-year plan that addresses your work life. What do you want to be doing three years from now? Where do you want to live? What income do you want to make? What do you want to learn? How do you want to grow?

Resources

Wellness Workbook, 148–64.

Bolles, R. *The Three Boxes of Life and How to Get Out of Them.* Berkeley, CA: Ten Speed Press, 1978.

——*What Color Is Your Parachute? A Practical Guide for Job-Hunters and Career-Changers.* Berkeley, CA: Ten Speed Press, Revised annually.

Covey, S. *The Seven Habits of Highly Effective People.* New York: Simon and Schuster, 1990.

Pelletier, K. *Healthy People in Unhealthy Places: Stress and Fitness at Work.* New York: Delacorte Press, 1984.

Sinetar, M. *Do What You Love, the Money Will Follow.* New York: Dell Publishing, 1989.

Stellman, J., and Henifin, M. *Office Work Can Be Dangerous To Your Health: A Handbook of Office Health and Safety Hazards and What You Can Do about Them.* New York: Pantheon Books, 1983.

···PROCESS 23· · · · · · · · · · · · · · · · · ·

Befriend the Earth

· · · · ·

*W*hen the air in cities becomes so toxic that allergic and sensitive individuals must wear masks and eye shields, there is trouble afoot. When major segments of a population can no longer trust the quality of the local water and resort to using their own filtration systems or buying bottled water, it's time for some serious reevaluation of priorities.

In Greek mythology, the earth was seen as mother and called "Gaia." The hypothesis that Gaia is a living entity, a single organism, was first suggested by Johannes Kepler hundreds of years ago. Recently that conception was developed further by James Lovelock in *A New Look at Life on Earth.* Observing that the planet has systems that regulate temperature, oxygen concentration, and other variables, he reasoned that the earth is much more than a hunk of rock with different species of plants and animals living on it. Rather it is a whole system made up of many smaller systems, including humankind.

There is no precise point at which the mind stops and the body starts. Similarly, there is no place where the individual stops and the environment starts, and vice versa. The accident at Chernobyl in the Soviet Union affected the agriculture of the entire continent of Europe. People no longer have the luxury of thinking of themselves as belonging to separate nations. Just as you cannot expect to find healthy fish in a polluted pond, you cannot expect to remain a healthy human being when you're breathing polluted air, eating devitalized food, and watching the earth being stripped of her resources. Wellness is an illusion without a commitment to the health of the whole planet.

DID YOU KNOW?

- If everyone in the US recycled one-tenth of the newspapers used, it would save 25 million trees a year.

- Every ton of recycled office paper saves 380 gallons of oil.

- All recycled glass is used to make more glass. Recycling glass instead of manufacturing new glass from sand reduces related air pollution by 20 percent and water pollution by 50 percent.

- Americans recycled 42.5 billion aluminum cans in 1988.

- If only 10 percent of the population purchased products with less plastic packaging 10 percent of the time, it would eliminate 144 million pounds of plastic from landfills and reduce industrial pollution from the manufacture of the packaging.

YOU CAN MAKE A DIFFERENCE

Contribute to a saner environment by examining your own lifestyle for waste. Start a family recycling program. Take the time to separate newspapers, glass, plastic, and metal items from your trash and send them to a local recycling center. Bring your own boxes or bags to the grocery store, buy in bulk, and buy foods and beverages in containers that can be recycled. Save and reuse mailing envelopes, boxes, packaging of all kinds, wrapping paper, aluminum foil, etc. Contribute clothing, old furniture, and household items to charitable organizations that distribute them or prepare them for resale.

There are many other practical, everyday choices you can make that will contribute to your own health and support the earth at the same time. You can:

- **Plant trees.** One million new urban trees would reduce CO_2 emissions in the US by 18 million tons and energy consumption by 40 billion kilowatt-hours (worth $4 billion) annually.

- **Eat lower on the food chain.** The reliance on meat and meat products in industrialized countries of the world is upsetting the entire world economy, necessitating the destruction of rain forests and farmlands to support the grazing of beef cattle.

- **Reflect on the interdependence of all things.** Realize that everything you think or say or do has an effect—either for good or ill—on your state of health and ultimately on the health of Gaia. Share what you know.

· · · · · · ·

*Nobody made a greater mistake
than he [sic] who did nothing because
he could only do a little.*

—EDMUND BURKE

· · · · · · ·

Resources

Wellness Workbook, 41–63, 165–84.

EarthWorks Group. *50 Simple Things You Can Do to Save the Earth.* Berkeley, CA: EarthWorks, 1989.

Lovelock, J. *Gaia: A New Look at Life on Earth.* New York: Oxford University Press, 1979.

MacEachern, D. *Save the Planet—750 Ways You Can Help Clean Up the Earth.* New York: Dell Publishing, 1990.

Robbins, J. *Diet for a New America.* Walpole, NH: Stillpoint Press, 1989.

Russell, P. *The Global Brain.* Los Angeles, CA: J. P. Tarcher, 1983.

Part IV

One Step Beyond

You've made it to the top of one peak and now you have the opportunity to survey what lies ahead or beyond. Part IV contains material of a more spiritual nature—processes that some may consider to be unconventional. These areas, in our view, are integral to the study of wellness since they touch upon essential human needs like inner peace and a sense of meaning. Welcome to the cutting edge of wellness, the edge of new possibilities for your own growth and healing.

The steps in Part IV include:

- using music to enhance your health
- cultivating silence for sanity
- spiritual dimensions of exercise
- self-forgiveness
- eating with awareness
- mental visualization for healing and stress management
- risk taking
- learning to live in the here and now
- making a friend of death

···PROCESS 24 ··················

Healing Music and Other Healthy Sounds

Without music life would be a mistake.
—NIETZSCHE

· · · · ·

In the Greek myth of Orpheus we find a powerful testimony to the power of music. Throughout his journey in the underworld, Orpehus played his lyre and sang. His music pacified the dark forces, bringing tears to the eyes of the gods and softening their hearts. Music does stir emotion. It is no wonder that it has been called the language of the soul. Music can soothe, or energize, or enervate, or fan the passions. You've no doubt experienced the emotional effects of music at some point in your life—perhaps at a wedding, a graduation, a funeral. In every culture, spiritual or religious ritual is accompanied by music, whether it involves the rousing drum beat of a tribal dance, the mournful strains of a medieval requiem, the awakening call of the cantor, or the joyous chorus of hand-clapping gospel singers.

Music alters the body and the mind. Just as loud, harsh sounds can cause injury to the eardrums and set the nervous system on edge, so, too, music and other sounds, like the ocean or your own heartbeat, can enhance deep relaxation, supply you with new energy, stimulate creativity, and even transport you into other states of consciousness. When used consciously, music is a form of healing. So, when you are particularly stressed, or feeling sick or in pain (with a backache, arthritis, or a bothersome cold, for instance), try using a little music therapy on yourself. Plants grow better with certain types of music. Why shouldn't the same be true for you?

LOSE YOURSELF IN MUSIC

The key to using music for healing is to allow yourself to get lost in it. Many people will listen to music critically, identifying the interactions of the various instruments or comparing the selection with other pieces. This is listening with the mind and does not promote relaxation, reverie, or emotional release. Therapeutic listening is done with the whole body. You literally drop your attention from your head to somewhere lower in your body—you imagine that your heart is listening; you allow your abdomen to be filled with the music; you let the music come in through your hands and feet; you breathe it. You keep letting go into the music, as if the sounds were waves or clouds that are carrying you away or supporting you.

Depending upon the type of music you choose, this method of listening can be either deeply relaxing or highly energizing. Listening with this degree of openness will alter the frequency of your brain waves, your rate of respiration, and your blood pressure. Imagery can be stimulated, memories evoked, emotions released, and tension dissipated.

Are you ready to give it a try? Pick out a piece of soothing music from your collection, or turn to the classical or "easy listening" station on your radio. When you find or hear something you like, sit back or lie down and close your eyes. Breathe. Allow your breath to carry the music deep within your body. Imagine that the music is playing from the inside out and "feel" it vibrate and move throughout your system. If there is an area of your body that is currently extra tense or in pain, let the music penetrate more deeply there. It takes just a little bit of imagination to do this. If at first you find difficulty with actually "feeling" it, simply narrate to yourself that this is happening. The more you do it, the more you will feel. When the piece is over, open your eyes and stretch. Notice how your body feels. Continue on your way.

Other Creative Uses of Sound for Wellness . . . .

• **Sing.** Open your mouth, your eyes, your throat. Sing at the top of your lungs, or quietly under your breath. Use singing to lift your spirits and to breathe more fully. Chant or hum. Use the repetition of the same sound or phrase to relax you, or to raise your consciousness, or to literally reprogram your body to a health–inspiring message.

- **Play an instrument.** Maybe it's time to dig out that old guitar, recorder, or drum, or to start taking lessons. Regina's husband, Jere, has recently taken to playing the harmonica—a skill he is learning from a simple book. For many people, music playing is both a form of energy release and relaxation, and a means of creative expression. Drums are particularly good for this and can be used without any instruction.

- **Listen to the movement of air** through your nostrils and to other natural sounds in the environment. Use wind sounds in combination with visualization to help you clear certain conditions—like headaches or a sense of confusion. Use water sounds for encouraging relaxation. The sounds of birds chirping is excellent for inspiring hope and joy. Be creative. Make up your own uses for natural sounds.

BUILD YOUR REPERTOIRE

Perhaps you have plenty of musical favorites to choose from already—different selections to help you to relax or to release built-up frustration. But if you don't, it may be time to start accumulating a music library of pieces that you can use for winding up or winding down. Many large music stores have a section of so-called new-age instrumental music where you can find many interesting selections. Classical music offers unending possibilities as well.

Resources

A catalogue of music listing selections for meditation and movement can be ordered by writing to Backroads Distributors, 417 Tamal Plaza, Corte Madera, CA 94925, or call them at 800-825-4848. Here are a few of our favorite musical selections to get you started.

CONTEMPORARY INSTRUMENTAL:

Enya. *Watermark*. Vocals with harp and synthesized accompaniment in two types: warm, nurturing callings-out to the heart and plucky, bouncy, make-your-body-move numbers. One selection, "Orinoco Flow," was a popular hit single in the late 1980s.

Kitaro. *Silk Road*. Melodic, hypnotic, soaring synthesizer sounds.

Lynch, Ray. *Sky of Mind*. A classic meditative piano and synthesizer album ideal for inward journeying.

Moffett, Karma. *Himalayan Bowls.* Random, an-melodic, bell-like oriental sounds. Deeply relaxing.

Morricone, Ennio. *The Mission* (sound track). Orchestral and choral—one of the all-time powerful albums for evoking emotions of all kinds.

Raphael. *Music to Disappear In.* Lush piano and synthesizer, perfect for when you feel like crawling back into the womb.

Tear of the Moon. Coyote Old Man Incan pan pipes and Native American flute. A meditative mood creator with simple, pure tones.

CLASSICAL:

Bach, The Six Brandenburg Concertos. Evoke a wide variety of feelings.

Beethoven, Symphony #6 in F, Opus 68 ("Pastoral"). Inspirational, soothing.

Mozart—almost anything, but Violin Concertos #3 and #5 are particularly magical and joyful.

Tchaikovsky, "Swan Lake" ballet suite and "Sleeping Beauty" ballet suite. Dance with your heart.

BOOKS:

Wellness Workbook, 60–63.

Campbell, D. *The Roar of Silence: The Healing Power of Breath, Tone, and Music.* Wheaton, IL: Theosophic Publishers, 1989.

Halpern, S. and Savary, L. *Sound Health—The Music and Sounds That Make Us Whole.* San Francisco, CA: Harper and Row, 1985.

··· PROCESS **25** ················

Cultivate Sanity through Silence

When real silence is dared, we can come very close to ourselves and to the deep center of the world.
—JAMES CARROLL

· · · · ·

*W*hen you need a quiet spot, it is rare to be able to find one free of noise from traffic, aircraft, office machinery, home appliances, TVs, or stereos. The noise pollution of modern society grows more strident every year. For many years, background noise in urban environments has been increasing at the rate of about a decibel per year, yet people rarely notice the increased noise because they have learned to block it out. But the stress it causes is not blocked. Besides the immediate danger of hearing loss due to long-term exposure to loud sounds, high levels of noise increase stress and irritability.

Rest and quiet are necessary when you are healing from illness, as well as when you simply want to renew yourself from the forces of overstimulation that are a part of life in the fast lane. It is important to find or create a place in which you can achieve some respite from noise, and to use that place for relaxation and healing, for creativity, and for contemplation or perhaps prayer. It is even more important to cultivate an interior silence—one that can be accessed even in the midst of the most distracting external noise. That's what meditation is all about. (See Process 11.)

Where or when can you experience silence? In a church, a library, in the middle of the night, in a wooded area, on a mountaintop, in your basement study? When was the last time you allowed yourself the gift of the sound of silence?

110

FEAR OF SILENCE

Many people experience great uneasiness when confronted with a lack of auditory input. Perhaps it is because silence forces them to think, to feel, to touch deep parts of themselves, to sense emptiness or meaninglessness. Learning to be comfortable with silence is really learning to be comfortable alone with yourself. It is one of the healthiest habits one can cultivate.

Nature isn't silent. Listen to the sounds of a stream or waterfall, the rush of the wind in the trees, the chirping of the birds. Yet nature is one of the greatest teachers of what real silence is about. Learning to be comfortable in nature, alone, without other forms of stimulation like music, hobbies, people to talk to, is the process of quieting the overactive mind and resting from the compulsiveness that drives life in these times.

. . . .

In the silence of the heart,
your inner voice can be heard.
With the silence of the mind,
the heart can speak its truth.

. . . .

Why not make a date with yourself in a quiet spot with nothing else to occupy you, and observe what happens.

Helpful Hints for a Quieter Home . . . .

At the very least, you can support yourself in a quieter home by eliminating some unnecessary noise. Here are some practical suggestions offered by the US Environmental Protection Agency (EPA):

- Compare, if possible, the noise output of different brands of appliances before making your selection.

- Use caution in buying children's toys that can make intensive or explosive sounds.

- Use a foam pad under blenders and mixers.

- Use carpeting to absorb noise, especially in areas where there is a lot of foot traffic.

- Hang heavy drapes over windows closest to outside noise sources.

- Put rubber or plastic treads on uncarpeted stairs. (They're safer, too.)

- Keep stereo and TV volume down and use headphones if others in the home want quiet.

- If you use a power mower or any other outdoor equipment, operate it at reasonable hours. The slower the engine setting, the quieter it will operate.

Resources

Wellness Workbook, 60–63.

Bloomfield, H. "The Healing Silence." In *Healers on Healing,* R. Carlson and B. Shield, eds. Los Angeles, CA: J. P. Tarcher, 1989.

Levine, S. A. *Gradual Awakening.* New York: Anchor/Doubleday, 1989.

Move Your Body/
Move Your Soul

*It is about 7:30 AM. I have been up since before
dawn. I have seen the world at its loveliest
moment. I have run more than eight miles, made
my body stronger, and enriched my soul. I will
shave, have a hot shower that will seem exotic and
sensual, eat, and be off to do what all of us do.
The difference is—I own the day.*
—JOEL HENNING, *Holistic Running.*

· · · · ·

$\mathcal{P}$rocess 15 dealt at length with the connection between wellness
and physical exercise. Now you get to move beyond the basics of exercising to consider movement in almost spiritual terms. When you think
of exercise, you probably think solely in terms of heart rates, strength,
and muscle tone. But because the body, mind, and soul are always
connected, exercising also involves your mind and your spirit. How you
move will affect how you think and feel about yourself, and vice versa.
And both will affect how you view life and the world in general. In
terms of your exercise programs, here's how it all connects.

• Keeping to a regular exercise program is a statement of personal power. It says that you are in charge of your own life, that you have
endurance, strength, flexibility, and determination. And these qualities will spill over into other domains of life and work. You can apply
your newfound endurance and flexibility to creative projects, to handling questions that arise in interpersonal relationships, to setting out
plans for the fulfillment of your dreams, and even to addressing ways
in which you can contribute to environmental concerns and world
issues.

- Regular exercise firms muscles, may help you shed pounds, and generally adds a healthy glow to the complexion. All of this can build a more positive self-concept. You like what you see and how you feel, and your sense of pride grows because of your commitment to yourself.

- When the body is tense or contracted, it colors the mind's perception of the world. Problems seem more problematical; deadlines more deadly. But a moving body is less likely to hold tension. A good run or a vigorous swim, for instance, can be ideal ways to release a dangerous build-up of worry. As Joel Henning said in the quote above, with exercise you get to "own the day."

- Exercise, like meditation, is a natural way of achieving an altered state of consciousness in which the rational and problem-oriented mind is temporarily put on hold. A deep sense of connectedness to all life and a sense of inner knowledge are among the benefits possible when exercise is used consciously.

- Exercising can actually be a form of prayer—a thanksgiving for the privilege of having a body and for simply being alive. When the whole body is used in this way, spirit becomes united with flesh; spirituality is grounded in the things of everyday life. Yoga, the martial arts, and some forms of dance specifically use the exterior posture to foster inner spiritual attitudes—such as serenity, gratitude, or one-pointedness. With practice, these exercise forms and the attitudes they foster insinuate themselves into all daily activities. You learn to cook your food, to drive to the office, and even to do your income taxes with the same degree of focus, thankfulness, and peace. Soon you are dancing through life, building the matrix for understanding, accepting, and participating in the great process of life. And out of that, purpose and meaning are created and revealed.

Now, or later today, use this experience as a way to move your body and refresh your soul:

1. Stand up, or remain seated if you wish, and breathe softly for a few moments. Put your palms together at the level of your chest, fingers pointing up in a traditional gesture of prayer. Reflect, for a moment or two, on the state of human beings in the world today.

2. Now raise your arms towards the sky, hands open and palms facing upwards. Raise your head and your eyes in the direction of your

hands. Think for a few moments about the "gifts from above"—the sun, the rain, the wind, etc.—that sustain life on planet Earth. Think about the future inhabitants of the earth and what is necessary for them.

3. Lower your arms now, palms facing the ground, head bowed. Remember the earth on which you reside, and reflect upon the "gifts from below"—the waters, the soil, the generative force. Remember your deceased relatives, your ancestors, all who have gone before. Repeat this sequence several times, remembering to breathe fully as you do so, and moving with as much smoothness and grace as possible each time. If you like you can add some appropriate music as background, or compose a chant, song, or prayer to accompany your movement. Let these movements develop into a dance. Conclude whenever you wish.

Resources

Wellness Workbook, 91–108.

MUSICAL ACCOMPANIMENT:

Pachelbel, Canon in D.

Any recording of Gregorian chants, Tibetan bells, or Native American songs.

See also the listings in Process 24.

Slow Down Your Fast Food

· · · · ·

*P*eople are eating out more frequently than ever before and much of that eating is done in fast-food restaurants. Eating on the run has become commonplace as the pace of life has quickened. It is not unusual to find people eating in their cars on the way to work, or between appointments, or combining their meals with important business meetings, the evening news, or a family argument.

WHAT'S THE PROBLEM?

- Fast eating can create indigestion, hiccups, intestinal pain, nausea, and sleepiness. A body that is under stress needs to work harder to digest food. When you do not chew your food adequately, you force the digestive system to work even harder.

- When you "stuff" your food and eat under pressure, or with distractions all around, you are less aware of what you are eating and of how the food feels in your body. Overeating is common since the food hasn't "landed" before you start loading in more.

- "Speed eating" exposes you to the risk of choking on your food. Death from choking is the fourth highest cause of accidental death in the US.

- You miss *life* when you miss appreciating the food that is right in your hands or in front of your eyes, nose, lips, teeth, and tongue. The faster you eat, the less you attend to what you are doing. The result is a lifestyle that is always six steps ahead of itself.

116

THE JOYS OF SLOWING DOWN

Food has aroma, and texture, and color, and form, and temperature, and weight both on the plate and in your mouth. Don't miss it. Somebody prepared the food you are eating. Somebody worked to purchase it. Somebody grew it. Somebody plowed the field. The soil nourished it. The sun supported it. And on and on. Eating is a way to appreciate the interdependence of living systems. When done with awareness, eating can inspire gratitude for more than simply the cessation of hunger.

To eat consciously (which generally means more slowly) with others is an act of communion with the rest of humanity. Food and eating together are core symbols in many religious traditions, and feasting has always been connected with celebrations of significance. To eat or drink together can be a way to seal a commitment. To share food with others is an expression of common necessity, as well as common potential.

The healthiest way to slow down speed eating is to start chewing, a long-forgotten activity in the repertoire of most modern people—adults as well as children. Walt Whitman once advised, "Drink your solids and chew your liquids." To "drink" solids is to chew them so well that they pass like liquids down your throat. To "chew" your liquids is to enjoy the sensation of them in your mouth. Chewing aids digestion because the saliva in the mouth initiates the breakdown of complex carbohydrates in the food. Chewing can also be an outlet for stress, a training of attention, and a means of strengthening the will. And that all adds up to increased patience and peace of mind.

THREE EXERCISES IN SLOW FOOD

• At your next meal, or next snack, pause for a moment before you start to eat. Reflect on all the work that went into producing the food you are about to eat; reflect with gratitude. Before you take your first bite, tune in all your senses. Take in the color and the aroma—and then really *taste* what you are eating. Roll the food on your tongue to get the full sense of its flavor and texture. Chew your first bite until it is liquified. Swallow. Then take a breath before you take your next bite. Continue eating at a more normal rate, this time noticing how much attention you generally give to your food, and how often you actually taste it. Start making a ritual of savoring at least the first bite of every meal and the first bite of every different type of food on your plate. You can do the same with a cup of tea or any other beverage as well. Bon appetit.

- Set up a special meal with friends. Create an atmosphere of elegant dining or ritual feasting, and make the presentation of the food so attractive that it encourages a slow savoring of every morsel.

- Once you get in the habit of slowing down your own eating and consciously enjoying your food it may be time to examine your life-style and that of your family for ways to generally decrease the stress associated with eating. In many homes the family meal is becoming a thing of the past. TV accompanies meals for many families, preoccupying attention and making conscious eating impossible. Perhaps it's time to turn off the TV and to reinstate the practice of a sit-down, family meal once a day, or once a week at least. Talk together about ways to make mealtimes more special and more restful for everyone.

Resources

Wellness Workbook, 64–90.

Sujata. *Beginning to See.* Berkeley, CA: Celestial Arts, 1987.

The Healing Power of Forgiveness

We must rid ourselves of the illusions, self-hate, and cynicism that ensue from futile expectations if we are to restore our vitality and hope to live well as real people in the real world. . . . To achieve true inner peace in our age of anxiety we must become increasingly aware of the flow and rhythm of our lives—who we are, our evolution and development, the time it takes for us to do things, our assets, limits, and tolerances.
—THEODORE ISAAC RUBIN, MD

· · · · ·

*A*ny program of self-change is bound to include some moments of discouragement. Disappointment and frustration are natural when the illusion of immediate results is broken, or the expectation of perfect discipline or consistency is not realized. It is easy to start off with a great burst of energy and then to slowly wind down. It is easy to set high initial goals and then have to reevaluate their feasibility. These are all normal turns in the cycle of change. They happen to everyone. The challenge is to deal realistically with these setbacks without allowing them to build into self-hatred or cynicism. That's why forgiveness is an integral part of the wellness journey.

There are times to be strict with yourself, and other times when easing up is necessary. Self-forgiveness is a way to handle disappointment and frustration and at the same time to keep moving ahead in your process of change. As you learn to practice self-forgiveness, which is self-acceptance, you naturally learn greater compassion for the shortcomings of others, and these traits keep you honest and flexible in your approach to life in general. This contributes greatly to your overall wellness.

THE HIGH PRICE OF "SHOULD"

Valuable life energy is wasted in burdening yourself with guilt and blame. (I should have done this . . . I shouldn't have done that . . .) These "shoulds" are danger signs if they are accompanied by feelings of self-hatred. Approach them cautiously, gently. They need to be examined to determine if they are just hangovers from early training ("You should always smile"), or if they are self-imposed demands and unrealistic beliefs that have no basis in current reality ("I should do everything perfectly or not at all"; "I should never let others see me as weak or they will take advantage of me").

Learning to observe yourself more honestly and then to practice forgiveness for all the ways you are not living up to your own expectations is a way of keeping well. With self-hatred you may build up an internal rigidity that is stressful on your system. Your emotional energy becomes toxic and that negativity weakens your immune system. With forgiveness you open yourself up again, letting energy flow more freely through the whole body, soothing emotions, and clearing the mind.

Many body-oriented therapies such as massage, rolfing, and bioenergetics, are designed specifically to help to release years of accumulated resentment and rigidity. Change is lasting and life-supporting only when it grows in soil that has been nourished with forgiveness. Without the compulsiveness of should's, changing can be a joyous adventure.

WHAT IS FORGIVENESS?

To forgive means to refuse to hold onto the past; to release grievance, recrimination, and blame; to reconcile. Realize, however, that we are not advocating resignation about your problems. Forgiveness and resignation are different things. Resignation is dry, passive, and lifeless. It is an attitude of defeat. Forgiveness is a choice—an active and lively process that requires your participation.

With forgiveness you willingly look below the surface of behaviors or feelings. Here you find the essence of yourself—the core of basic goodness that may have been temporarily obscured but never diminished. When you connect with yourself (or others) and acknowledge what you find, forgiveness is so much easier.

Forgiveness of yourself or others often brings with it a relaxation in the body and peace of mind. This harmony is the essence of healing and the heart of wellness.

A Short Course on Forgiveness . . . .

1. Reflect on one or two ways in which you are hard on yourself. What do you blame yourself for? What do you feel bad or guilty about? What "mistake" of your recent past still burdens you with feelings of inadequacy or regret? Write it down here. For example:

   I feel bad about overeating at almost every meal.

2. Identify the message(s) of self-hatred, the judgements, the interpretations, that accompany this activity or omission. Record those here. For example:

   The messages I tell myself about my overeating are: "I'm undisciplined, weak, and lazy."

3. Ask yourself if you would really like to do something to change that behavior or problem. If the answer is yes, the most effective change will take place if you simultaneously forgive yourself. Go on to step 4. If the answer is no or maybe, read ahead anyway. It is important to be able to accept yourself as much when you are saying no as when you are saying yes.

4. The secret key to forgiveness is the intention to forgive. Forgiveness is not a feeling, so if you wait for your feelings to magically change, you will probably wait forever. Forgiveness is a decision. And it is followed by the willingness and the effort to act on the basis of what you have decided. Quite simply, you make the intention to forgive, exert some effort in acting differently, watch as you fall short of your goal, day after day, and then you make the intention again.

   Be patient. Your willingness to forgive yourself is a monumental step. The renewed intention to forgive will begin to change your mental programming and to build the energy for spontaneous action. Soon the changes will come.

State your intention now. "I forgive you, _____ , (your name) for _____ (the thing you want to forgive). I release you from any guilt or blame, now and forever." Use this statement frequently throughout your day.

The exercises below will also help you to focus your awareness on forgiveness. Experiment with them.

- Forgive by grieving your loss. You may not be able to forgive if you have not adequately mourned a loss. For instance, when people cut down on or eliminate smoking, they give up many patterns that were sources of strokes for them (see Process 4), like their daily conversations with fellow smokers. Ask yourself: What have I lost in my situation? For the time being, forget about trying to forgive yourself and concentrate on telling the story of your pain or problem to every willing ear. Find friends who are not afraid of strong emotions and cry with them. Write letters to yourself or to others, describing and lamenting your loss. Enlist the help of a support group or seek professional counseling to work out your grief. This is hard work, so don't give up too soon.

- Close your eyes and repeat your own name, gently, as if you were talking to a lover. Then picture yourself in your own mind's eye. Imagine that you are surrounded by a warm, golden light. Let your breathing deepen and imagine that light growing brighter. Pretend that the light is melting you, layer by layer, revealing your inner fears and pain, and finally revealing the loving core of your being—your hunger for happiness, love, and peace for yourself and others. Keep this picture in your mind for a few minutes. Allow forgiveness to enter in. Speak words of acceptance and acknowledgement to yourself. Open your eyes.

- Lack of forgiveness may be a failure to appreciate the beauty and strength of who you really are. Focusing on these qualities in yourself is helpful in practicing forgiveness. Make a list of all the things that are great about you. Include your talents, accomplishments, sensitivities, caring and generous activities, courage, or other virtues—anything you can think of. Don't be satisfied until you have a good long list. Read it over. Read it over again.

. . . .

THE SERENITY PRAYER
God grant me the serenity
to accept the things I cannot change,
The courage to change the things I can,
And the wisdom to know the difference.

—ANONYMOUS

. . . .

Resources

Wellness Workbook, 14–22.

Bradshaw, J. *Healing the Shame That Binds You.* Deerfield Beach, FL: Health Communications, 1988.

Rubin, T. I. *Reconciliations: Inner Peace in an Age of Anxiety.* New York: Berkeley Books, 1980.

A Course in Miracles. Tiburon, CA: Foundation for Inner Peace, 1975.

Put Yourself in the Picture— of Health

What you see is what you get.

· · · · ·

$\mathcal{H}$umans are image-making creatures. As we considered previously (see Process 7), even without knowing it, you are making mental pictures constantly. As someone gives you directions, you visualize the route. As you read about a place you have never been, you create images of the surroundings. Even though you may never have seen a gallstone or a tumor, the words themselves suggest an image to your mind.

The interesting thing about images is that, somewhat like words, they create emotional states which affect brain chemistry, and brain chemistry will depress or strengthen every system in the body, including the immune system. It pays to know what types of imagery you are currently generating and how to make that imagery work for you. It is a powerful tool for personal wellness.

In biofeedback training, for example, people learn to lower their blood pressure by imagining vapors rising from a sun-warmed lake. They can also learn to significantly raise their hand temperature by creating a mental picture that their hands are being warmed by the sun, or are immersed in warm water. Raising hand temperature has certain health benefits. For instance, it is correlated with a decrease in headache pain.

Since the early 1970s, Carl Simonton, MD, and his colleagues have been successfully using visualizations along with conventional therapies to induce remissions and even cure cancer. Patients are taught to combine periodic relaxation with visualizations of healthy, energetic cells fighting and destroying the weaker and disorganized cancer cells.

Visualization skills are being taught to business executives to help them expand their creative thinking and to create mental pictures of the goals they want to accomplish. With athletes, visualization is used in conjunction with physical practice to refine performance and build self-confidence. In childbirth, visualization allows a woman to remain relaxed and focused during labor. And with patients anticipating surgery, it helps to calm fears by giving the patient some sense of control over their own internal states. Visualization is growing in popularity because it works.

Imagery Experience 1—Paint a Picture of Health for Yourself

Read this over and then guide yourself through it, or ask a friend to read it slowly to you, as you follow the steps.

1. Take a moment to relax. Breathe deeply and let your body sink into your chair. Close your eyes. Now recall a time in your life when you felt great, when your body was as healthy as it could be. Imagine yourself doing something in that healthy state—like taking a walk or dancing.
2. Notice how you are dressed in your mental picture. What does your complexion look like? How does your energy level feel? The trick here is to use as many sensory pathways as possible to reinforce that picture of health. Notice the smile on your face. Breathe.
3. Identify with that picture for a few minutes. With your breath, draw in that image so that it penetrates deep within your body. Let yourself experience the same degree of energy and feeling of aliveness that you have in the image. Continue to hold that image for a minute if possible.
4. Now open your eyes. How do you feel?

This exercise is a good beginning, a way to practice developing and actually feeling the effects of healing imagery. As you begin to be at ease with the process, you can use it to help alleviate the tension and discomfort associated with a variety of symptoms, such as nausea, headache, muscle pain. The next exercise will show you how.

Imagery Experience 2—An Imaging Flip for Symptom Relief

Your mental images may be keeping you stuck in pain, in tension, in depression. But they can be "flipped over" to become healing images, and thus used to alleviate the same pain, tension, or depression.

Here, as above, read over the whole exercise for yourself first, or ask a friend to read it to you as you follow the steps.

125

1. Focus on one problem area. Perhaps it is the chronic tension in your right shoulder, or the nausea you experience riding in a car or plane. (Even if you are not experiencing that pain or tension now, you can use this exercise to prepare a healing image that will be available to you when you need it.) Note as many sensory aspects of this condition as you can. This will help you to create the healing image. Ask yourself:

   a. Is there a picture associated with the problem or pain? (For instance, tight, knotted nautical ropes, or a murky, stagnant pool.)

   b. Is there a sound connected with the problem or pain? (For instance, a grinding or gurgling sound.)

   c. Is there a texture associated with it? (A sore throat, for instance, might feel like rough sandpaper; an upset stomach might feel slimy.)

   d. Is there a temperature associated with it? (A headache might feel hot; a broken arm might feel cold.)

   e Is there a smell or taste associated with it?

   f. Is there a movement associated with it? (Churning, pounding, stabbing?)

2. Now for the "flipping" part. The essential question here is what the problem or pain look, feel, smell, sound, taste like *when it is alleviated or cured*. For the image you have of the condition, substitute its opposite. For instance:

   — Knotted ropes are slowly untied and loosely laid out on the deck.

   — A stagnant pool is drained and filled with clear, sweet water.

   — A dark cloud of pain in the head is penetrated with sunlight.

   — A pounding sound is replaced by the sound of a waterfall.

3. Now, relax. Take a few slow, deep breaths and recall the healing image you have just created. Use words if necessary to reinforce the image. For instance: "My head is filled with billowy, white clouds." Continue to rest for at least 5 or 10 mintues (more if possible) as you hold the healing image in your mind's eye. As your mind wanders or you are distracted by your pain, gently recall the healing image once again. Continue to use slow, gentle breathing to deepen your relaxation.

Don't be discouraged if you can't conjure up all the images we have suggested. Use the ones that are strongest for you. Be patient with yourself in anticipating results, but know that other people have used this exercise to great advantage. Give it a try.

Imagery Experience 3—Making Your Dreams Come True. . .

Look back to the beginning of this book where you designed a few specific goals for yourself as you began. Choose one of your primary goals and use imagery to form a picture of yourself with that goal already accomplished. For instance, if you are working to relieve back-ache, create, in your mind's eye, a picture of yourself moving around your house, or walking, or dancing easefully, without pain. Many people will enhance this approach by making a collage of magazine pictures, all indicating the positive outcome of their desired goal. By posting this collage somewhere that you will see it often, you will be inspired again to orient yourself towards its accomplishment.

Resources

Wellness Workbook, 128–47.

Achterberg, J. *Imagery in Healing.* Boston, MA: Shambhala, 1985.

Gawain, S. *Creative Visualization.* New York: Bantam Books, 1982.

Simonton, C., Matthews-Simonton, S., Creighton, J. *Getting Well Again.* Los Angeles, CA: J.P. Tarcher, 1978.

···PROCESS 30 ·····················

Don't Play It Safe

The first step . . . shall be to lose the way.
—GALWAY KINNELL

· · · · ·

*D*on't get the wrong idea! This is not a plea for foolhardiness but rather an invitation to challenge yourself to express more of your tremendous potential. To do that you need to cultivate stress up to a point, and you need to develop appreciation for the lessons and potential growth that disease or problems will afford you.

Having come this far in the book, you probably have the impression that stress and disease are enemies and that your job is to eliminate them from the face of the earth. But that is not so. Stress is necessary for life. Without it you'd be slithering on the ground instead of walking upright. Without it you'd be dead! Illness is not necessarily bad, either. In fact, it is a virtually unavoidable fact of life, and the sooner you accept it as a friend and teacher, the better off you will be.

This process is an invitation into greater risk taking—the kind that stretches you beyond your limited definitions of yourself and your definitions of what is possible. The great adventure of life is to commit yourself to something impossible, something that exceeds your grasp, something that cannot be accomplished in your lifetime. As Woody Allen has said, in so many words, if you aren't making any mistakes, or if people aren't criticizing you, you probably aren't taking any risks. You probably aren't having any fun, and you certainly aren't living/ growing into your fullest potential.

Health is a function of participation in life. Those who attempt to play it too safe often end up lonely, isolated from others, or obsessed with their own health issues. These attitudes limit one's world, and weaken the immune system as well. How about it? When was the last time you took a risk? did something uncharacteristic? committed yourself to a great task?

128

Here are a few simple suggestions to help keep life "unsafe":

Avoid the well-balanced life. Life that is perfectly balanced is safe, limited, homogenized, and boring. Any programs that promise complete harmony are sure setups for failure and disappointment.

Cultivate chaos. Without chaos the possibility of serendipity is ruled out. Operate without usual rules and schedules for a day or two and refuse to make it a problem. Let things break down and don't fix them: then deal with the consequences. Learn what happens.

Think stress. Become a person of inner strength by cultivating situations that tax your courage, discipline, and commitment. If you've got a problem that you think is big or important, give yourself a bigger problem by taking on a commitment to a task "bigger than you are." Now watch the first problem fall into place. And don't be fooled by thinking that it necessarily means you will have to work harder. The point is that busy, committed people quickly learn to work smarter!

Resist comfort. Avoid the numbing effects of a "walking death" by keeping an edge of discomfort for yourself. If you run for a sweater every time you're cold, or turn up the air conditioner every time you're hot, you keep yourself insulated in more ways than one. Appreciate unavoidable pain and use it as a way to learn what stuff you're made of. Remedies that mask symptoms also mask the information that those symptoms might afford.

"Pig out." The healthier your diet, the more important it is to indulge yourself, occasionally, with all the foods you think are so "bad" for you (unless you are actually allergic to them).

Put on some rock and roll music, pump up the volume, and dance!

Don't be nice. Be simple. Be straightforward. Be caring. Be daring. Be wild. Be silly. Be uncharacteristic. Be anything. . . but don't be N-I-C-E. Not all the time. You know what we mean? Yes, nice is a four-letter word.

Apprentice yourself to greatness. There is nothing harder yet ultimately more satisfying than being stretched beyond the limited vision you have for yourself. Stay around people who provoke you to greatness, who keep you uncomfortable, who ask more of you than you think is possible. Study what they have to teach you.

Live your questions. It is a natural human phenomenon that we tend to find or see what we are looking for, and to overlook or miss what we haven't anticipated. Our thoughts, and in this case our questions, will therefore "mold" our experience of reality. (For example, if you are fascinated by the nature and meaning of time, your questioning will motivate and even direct you into situations where you will learn about it.) It is important to cultivate questions that are open-ended in order to live in an open-ended world. Otherwise we mold our world into black and white, and answer all questions with right or wrong— yes or no.

. . . .

Be patient toward all that is unsolved in your heart and try to love the questions themselves . . . the point is to live everything. Live the questions now. Perhaps you will then gradually, without noticing it, live along some distant day into the answer.

—Rainer Maria Rilke, *Letters to a Young Poet*

. . . .

Right now: List some of the ways in which you currently "play it safe" in your life. Determine one rule you're willing to break and do it.

Resources

Kriegel, R. and Kriegel, M. *The C Zone: Peak Performance Under Pressure.* Garden City, NY: Doubleday, 1984.

Van Oeck, R. *A Whack on the Side of the Head: How to Unlock Your Mind for Innovation.* New York: Warner Books, 1983.

Be Here Now

> *The past is dead. The future is imaginary.*
> *Happiness can only be in the Eternal, Now Moment.*
> —KEN KEYES

· · · · ·

The philosophy of taking one day at a time is a healthy one. When you live in either the past or the future, you miss what is going on right in front of your nose. When you are going through hard times, the habit of living essentially in the present, one day at a time, or even one hour at a time, can literally mean the difference between breakdown and sanity. It can help you endure a seemingly unbearable situation and find meaning in the simplest things, even when circumstances appear hopeless.

Meanings constantly change because your life is constantly changing. The ring that you wore yesterday and treasured as a sign of eternal fidelity may be tarnishing in the back of your kitchen drawer tomorrow. Meanings are found in the present. Looking to the future for happiness or living on past glories is a sure setup for disappointment and a way to lose touch with what is most wanted and needed to support your wellness today.

Life is less satisfactory when it is lived only in a linear mode— constantly moving along a line that extends into the future, piling one experience upon another. It's a little like being a tourist in a great museum trying to see everything in a few hours. But fortunately there is another dimension to life—the round dimension of living in and savoring the present moment. Poets and songwriters have struggled for ages to express this reality. "Today is the first day of the rest of your life" and other memorable quotes remind us to appreciate *what is*. Mystics and spiritual teachers have assured us of the same thing. Jesus said, "So, do not worry about tomorrow" (Matt. 6:34). Sufi master Meher Baba continually reminded his friends, "Don't worry, be happy," an exhortation that was turned into a hit song in the late 1980s.

Ways to Stay Here and Now . . . .

- Use your breath as a cue to remain present and receptive to all sensations—sights, smells, sounds, textures—and the many possibilities that each moment offers.

- Stop before every meal or each new task. Pray or reflect about what you are about to do so that you don't miss it.

. . . .

*Normally we do not so much
look at things as overlook them.*

—ALAN WATTS

. . . .

- Live one day at a time. Limit your worries to this day, at the very most. The quality of each day can always be upgraded by remembering how precious time is.

- Make a series of signs or pictures that you post around your house, in your office, in your car. Let each sign say something or depict something to remind you to *be present,* now.

- Take time each day for silence and solitude. The simple practice of meditation or focused consciousness is the most powerful means of moving into the here and now and staying there more consistently.

- Exercise vigorously and regularly. Using your body in this way can be a natural high—a means of altering your consciousness, and a powerful way to connect with the multisensory experience of life in the present moment.

Right now: Look at your hands. Don't just glance at them; examine them at length. Discover something about your hands that you hadn't known or noticed before. Now touch your own hands. Explore them and the many different ways to contact and move them. Feel them against your face. Smell them. Taste them. Sit and rest and look deeply at your hands as if they were your most precious friends. For the rest of this day, whenever you notice or think about your hands, let them remind you to breathe and relax into the present moment.

Resources

Wellness Workbook, 196–207.

Dass, R. *Be Here Now.* New York: Crown Publishing, 1971.

Keyes, K. *Handbook to Higher Consciousness.* Coos Bay, OR: Living Love
Publications, 1975.

Make a Friend of Death

We are all terminal.

· · · · ·

$\mathcal{T}$he recognition of mortality gives impetus to life in a way that almost nothing else can. It urges you on to make more constructive use of your time and can help you to keep your priorities in order. From the perspective of your deathbed, things that are troubling you now might seem trivial and nonproblematical. If you lived more consistently with the realization of death as a fact of life you might live more sensuously and intensely. The Buddha, Siddartha, started on his path to understanding and enlightenment when he first saw a dead body. It plunged him into deep reflection on the meaning of life.

With death as your friend, your might also live more consciously—caring for your health and well-being, honoring your body as the only one you've got. You might live more playfully—taking more risks and not taking yourself so seriously, playing life as a game! It is paradoxical that befriending death is a way of increasing your joy in life. You might live with more ecological awareness—realizing that your life and health, and that of your children, depends upon the life and health of this planetary body, Earth.

When you think about it, you are always "dying" in some tiny ways every day, because you are always in the process of change. Change means saying good-bye to something in order to say hello to something else. Each good-bye is a little death. Baby teeth fall out, adult teeth move up. Skin cells die and are sloughed off as new skin replaces it. A new job means death to the previous one. Growing means dying to old patterns of belief.

Every moment you are being born to something new, dying to something old. Nothing lasts. As you become more aware of death and rebirth in each moment, you constantly reevaluate priorities. You can learn to treasure the transformative quality and possibility of each death and each birth. You can remember to celebrate the process of life instead of wasting valuable energy in ongoing resistance.

In the traditions of some North American tribes, a death chant is learned early in life—a particular repetition of words that serves to remind the young men and women of their destiny and to help them prepare for it throughout their lives. Whenever they are in danger, or ill, or frightened, the death chant is recalled. It actually becomes a source of reassurance, something that builds strength.

- Look around you. Imagine that this is going to be the last day of your life. Don't just skim over the thought, let it sink in, as if you were an actor who had to feel it in order to play an important part. Think about how you would like to reorient your attitudes and your tasks to accommodate what you know is going to happen. Would you work differently? Would you relate to people differently? How do your big problems look from this perspective? Is there a person you want to contact to make peace with? Is there a letter that needs to be written? Have you made out a will? Well, what are you waiting for? Do one thing to support your new view of your life.

- Make a list of the things you fear about death. It might include: the possibility of pain, being a burden to others, the hardship and sorrow that your death will be to your family, the sense of incompleteness, the feeling that you didn't do all you intended to do with your life, a sense of meaninglessness, that you never found your purpose, etc.

Now ask yourself, How do these fears reflect upon the ways in which I live, or fail to live, my life now? What do my fears of death tell me about my real fears of life?

This is a valuable exercise to go through together with other members of your family or with friends. Talking about death allows people to share some of their deepest feelings or at least opens the door to that. It is healthier to face your fears rather than spending your precious life trying to hide from them.

Resources

Wellness Workbook, 196–207.

Castenada, C. *Journey to Ixtlan.* New York: Pocket Books, 1972.

————*The Power of Silence.* New York: Simon and Shuster, 1987.

Levine, S. *Healing Into Life and Death.* Garden City, NY: Doubleday, 1987

Neale, R. *The Art of Dying.* New York: Harper and Row, 1973.

· · ·Conclusion· ·

· · · · ·

*C*ongratulations! You've reached the end of the book! By what ever means you arrived here—having gone step-by-step, from beginning to end, or having skipped through, stopping only to address your most pressing needs—we hope that the small changes you've made have begun to make a difference in your life. We hope too, that you are experiencing increased self-awareness and self-appreciation, that you have a sense of greater inner strength, and, above all, that you are living more well.

We began by comparing the wellness process to a journey. Our intention was to start you off on the path and to stay with you as long as needed. At this point you have several options. You could circle back to review Processes 1 and 2, evaluate your growth, and set some new goals. If there were processes you passed over earlier, you could explore them now or you could delve further into any area, using the resources listed. The *Wellness Workbook*, for instance, could be your next challenge. (You could begin by reading the three appendices to this book, as they contain certain key material drawn from the *Wellness Workbook*.)

Whatever you do, don't stop now, because wellness is not a project to be completed and hung on the wall for display. It is an ongoing life process, a journey without end. So take advantage of the momentum you have now and continue on your way.

What Next? ·

Why not take a few moments now to summarize your learning here. Using each of the unfinished sentences listed below, write as many responses to each one as you wish—the more the better.

As a result of working with this book I have learned . . .

With regard to using this book I am proud that . . .

With regard to using this book I am disappointed that . . .

To support my wellness I want to . . .

To support my wellness I need to . . .

To support my wellness I will . . .

The Iceberg Model

· · · · ·

$\mathcal{A}$s you work through the processes contained in this book it may help to consider the unseen realms that largely underlie the state of your wellness.

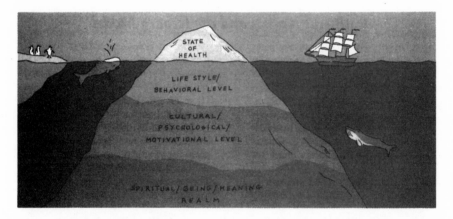

Illness and health are only the tip of the iceberg. To understand their causes, you must look below the surface.

Icebergs are interesting! They reveal only about one-tenth of their mass above the water. The remaining nine-tenths remain submerged. This is why they are such a nightmare in navigation; and why they make such an appropriate metaphor in considering your state of wellness.

Your current state of health—be it one of disease, or vitality—is just like the tip of the iceberg. This is the apparent part—what shows. If you don't like it, you can attempt to change it, "do things" to it, chisel away at an unwanted condition. But, whenever you knock some off, more of the same comes up to take its place.

To understand all that creates and supports your current state of health, you have to look "underwater." The first level you encounter is the Lifestyle/Behavioral level—what you eat, how you use and exercise your body, how you relax and let go of stress, and how you safeguard yourself from the hazards around you.

Many people follow lifestyles that they know are destructive, both to their own well-being and to that of our planet. Yet, they may feel powerless to change them. To understand why, you must look still deeper, to the Psychological/Motivational level. Here you find out what moves people to lead the lifestyles they have chosen. There are payoffs we get from being overweight, smoking, driving recklessly. There are different payoffs from eating well, being considerate of others, and getting regular exercise.

The norms of the culture you live in powerfully affect your daily thoughts and habits—often consciously in subtle or insidious ways. Cultural norms, combined with the long-lasting effects of dysfunctional childhood experiences (e.g., growing up in a family where emotions were suppressed or overly expressed), serve to keep people on "automatic," repeating self-destructive patterns for a lifetime. You can break out of these cycles by reevaluating all the parts of the environment you create around you—friends, workplace, home—and making the appropriate changes.

Exploring below the Psychological/Motivational level, we encounter the Spiritual/Being/Meaning level. Other descriptors here may include: transpersonal, philosophical, or metaphysical. Actually, we prefer to call it a realm rather than a level because it has no clear boundaries. It includes the mystical and mysterious, and everything else in the unconscious mind, and concerns such issues as your reason for being, the real meaning of your life, or your place in the universe. How you address these questions, and the answers you choose, underlie and permeate all of the layers above. Ultimately, this realm determines whether the tip of the iceberg, representing your state of health, is one of disease or wellness.

Reprinted from Travis, J. and Ryan, R. *Wellness Workbook*.

The Wellness Energy System

*As a human being you are an energy transformer,
connected with the whole universe. The condition
of each of your life processes, including the illness
and wellness processes, depends on how you
manage energy.*

· · · · ·

$\mathcal{E}$verything is energy—including the paper in your hands and the thoughts you are now thinking as you read this. Your body/mind/spirit is a sophisticated *energy transformation system.*

You *take in* energy from all the sources around you—in the form of such tangible inputs as air, food, heat, light, sound, and physical touch, and less tangible emotional/spiritual inputs as attention, caring, love, enthusiasm, and extrasensory data.

You *organize* and *transform* that energy—some for internal "house-keeping" (digestion, circulation, and neural activity), some for tissue repair, and some for the generation of emotions and thinking processes, including spiritual insights and altered states of consciousness.

You *return* some of the energy to the environment around you in other forms—for instance, as heat, carbon dioxide, and other products. You also return energy through communication and physical work, and through the expression of emotions and creativity.

ILLNESS AND ENERGY

When the flow of energy in your system is balanced and smooth, you feel good. When there is interference in the flow, illness is often the result. Interference can occur at any point. It could be due to:

141

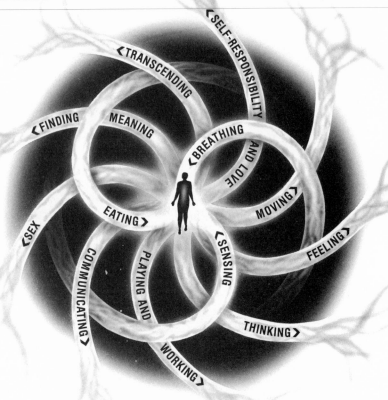

The Wellness Energy System has twelve components—three are the major sources of energy input: eating, breathing, and sensing; and nine are forms of energy output: self-responsibility and love, moving, feeling, communicating, thinking, sex, working and playing, finding meaning, and transcending.*

- low-quality or insufficient input energy—such as polluted air or a poorly balanced diet

- an insufficient or weak transformer—such as a damaged heart or an overweight body

- blockages to output energy—such as the inability to express emotions or no one to communicate with

The challenge of being well, then, is the challenge of maximizing the efficiency of this energy transformation system.

*From Travis, J. and Ryan, R. *Wellness Workbook.* First developed by John in 1976, The Wellness Energy System is the theoretical framework for both this book and the *Wellness Workbook.*

Cultural Norms and Wellness

· · · · ·

Cultural norms are the beliefs and values generally accepted by a population. Your culture's norms guide everything from your sexual behavior to the career path you choose to what you eat for breakfast. Cultural norms either encourage or undermine health and wellness. In recent years the cultural norms for jogging and other forms of solitary exercise have changed dramatically, as have the cultural norms for the acceptance of smoking, especially in public places.

Researchers have found that norms themselves usually lag years behind what the majority of people privately think or even practice. This "lowest common denominator" effect serves to maintain the public mind at a level of acceptance that encompasses the total population even if most people actually think the behavior is outmoded and inadequate.

HOW CULTURAL NORMS ARE CHANGED

Cultural norms change when enough individuals adopt a particular change within their own lifestyles. It then becomes economically and politically expedient to provide programs, legislation, or products that support the changes.

It is important, therefore, not to underestimate the power of one person to make a difference. Just as your personal wellness process can begin with small changes in your lifestyle, so too can these small changes help to alter cultural norms. And you bring about these changes just as you bring about changes in yourself.

REGINA SARA RYAN lives in Prescott, Arizona, where she teaches courses in human development at Prescott College. When she isn't writing or teaching, Regina performs with the Baul Theatre Company, a transformational theatre group in Prescott, and travels in the US and Europe with her friends in LGB, a rock n' roll band.

JOHN W. TRAVIS, MD, MPH, completed his medical training in Boston and a General Preventive Medicine residency at Johns Hopkins. In 1975 he gave up the practice of sick care to found the pioneering Wellness Resource Center. He and his wife/partner Meryn Callander are forming a small community for helping professionals interested in simple, cooperative living in the hills of Northern California.

WHAT IS WELLNESS ASSOCIATES?

Wellness Associates is a nonprofit educational organization dedicated to enhancing personal and planetary well-being. It evolved from the world's first wellness center, which was founded by John in 1975. It distributes the *Wellness Workbook, Wellness for Helping Professionals,* and the *Wellness Inventory* throughout the world, as well as facilitating seminars in CultureMaking* for small circles of helping professionals. For more information write Box 5433-J, Mill Valley, CA 94942.

---

*CultureMaking is the art of shifting the cultural norms of dominance and power-over to those of partnership and cooperation—through both inner work on self-worth and the creating of compassionate cultures—at home and on the planet.

Your feedback and comments are invaluable to us.
Please share your thoughts and feelings
about the book below, and mail to:

Wellness Associates, Box 5433-J, Mill Valley, CA 94942

Dear Regina and John:

SPECIAL OFFER

If you liked this book and want to learn more about wellness, you can order the *Wellness Workbook* from us for $13.95 postpaid. If you fill out the feedback page on the opposite side of this foorder form, we'll include—at no extra charge—one copy each of the *Wellness Inventory* and the *Global Wellness Inventory*. You can also order either Wellness Inventory separately

Please send me

_____ copies of the *Wellness Workbook* at $13.95   _____

_____ copies of the *Wellness Inventory* at $1.95 each   _____

_____ copies of the *Global Wellness Inventory* at $1.95 each   _____

_____ copies of *Wellness for Helping Professionals* at $24.95 each   _____

more information on the above titles

California residents add local sales tax

I am enclosing payment by ☐ check or money order
☐ VISA   ☐ Mastercard

Credit card # ($15 minimum) _____
Expiration date _____

Ship to: _____

_____

_____

_____

City _____ State ____ Zip _____

Send your order to:
Wellness Associates, Box 5433-J, Mill Valley, CA 94942